Breaking Your Bubble

Breaking Your Bubble

Return to Your Natural Design by Integrating Ancient Wisdom and Modern Science for True Health

Razvan Balotescu, MD

Hardcover Edition
ISBN: 978-1-7349792-4-4

Publisher: Visual Reflex LLC
Enroll for the newsletter at www.razvanbalotescu.com

Table of Contents

For my patients.

Preface

This book offers a unique approach to enhancing your well-being. It focuses on realigning your lifestyle to your natural design and enhancing your body's natural healing capacities, reducing the need for long-term medication use.

If you have a chronic condition, you can follow the three steps below to improve it. If you are healthy and just want to improve your well-being, you may skip the first step.

1. **Identify, understand, and remove or reduce the possible or probable root causes of your condition.** The causes of most chronic conditions fall into two categories:

    -   *underlying causes*, usually indolent, persistent, and subtle, like genetic predispositions, previous injuries, or persisting aggressions. Examples of persisting aggressions are long-term exposure to harmful chemical or biological agents, bad habits, or the absence of good habits. These underlying causes are often mixed, combined, and of different degrees of importance. They often produce low-grade, hard-to-detect inflammation, and subtle or no symptoms. They respond slowly to treatment. Look for any abnormalities in medical tests, imaging, or other laboratories that would provide more information, but conventional tests are usually normal. Some serious conditions like cancer, heart attack, or stroke represent the tip of the iceberg of the underlying damages created by these persisting indolent causes. See Chapters 1, 2, and 13.

- *triggers or exacerbating factors*, usually manifesting repetitive, acute, or subacute as digestive symptoms like heartburn, back pain without a serious trauma, a persisting cough, or uncontrolled high blood pressure. Often, the symptoms resolve or improve with treatment but keep coming back. The triggers are apparent and temporary: high stress, food or environment irritants, and the resulting symptoms respond to conventional treatment. They push us over the edge as they exacerbate the underlying chronic condition. Conventional tests are often abnormal and help to identify them. See Chapter 13.

2. **Increase your body's resilience and recovery capacity.** This works preventively or curatively by removing unhealthy habits and introducing good ones. One of the most effective ways is to go into "survival mode" and embrace healthy, natural challenges by regularly practicing any or all of the three old lifestyle activities—fasting, cold plunges, and exercise. The goal is to realign your lifestyle with your inherited natural design. You need to implement other important changes to align with this concept, like adding minerals to your drinking water, correcting the way you sit, or eating locally and in season. See Chapters 1 through 6.

3. **Align your life to healthy and constructive higher purposes.** Our natural propensity for abuse and damaging ourselves and others is a significant source of unnecessary suffering. It affects not only emotional

health but also physical and spiritual health. Hoping and fighting to achieve higher creative purposes will mobilize your almost unlimited resources, providing you with strength and good health. See Chapters 12 and 14 through 17.

To achieve a state of joy and well-being, we also need healthy and stable relationships between our family members and in our social circles. We need to embrace our predecessors' values and wisdom, which have stood the test of time and brought us success, peace, and prosperity.

But now, particularly in the last decade, Western values are in danger from the new culture and ideology that take advantage of our abusive nature and create racial, social, and ethnic conflicts. The significant and harmful changes in our contemporary society stem mostly from an unprecedented restructuring of the world power system enabled by advancing technologies. These changes are profound, ignore our natural design, and affect our health at all levels, physical, emotional, and socio-cultural. An unprecedented alliance has formed between large, powerful, multi-billion dollar corporations and governments, leading to an unparalleled concentration of power and control in the hands of a few. This new toxic cultural bubble is resetting our values, meanings, and purposes, inflicting chaos, destruction, and damage to our well-being. See Chapter 17.

About the Author

Born and raised in communist Romania, I came to the United States at 24, seeking freedom, opportunities, and stability. After medical school, I completed my Internal Medicine Residency at a Yale-affiliated program in Danbury, Connecticut, and have over twenty-five years of experience in internal medicine.

As a primary care physician, I have had the privilege of exploring the intricate connections between physical, emotional, and spiritual factors in patient care. I came to understand that many health issues are avoidable, self-induced, and unnecessary, driven by the complexities of human nature. Consequently, in my private practice, I have focused on lifestyle, disease prevention, and minimizing long-term prescription medications.

My fascination with human nature and its connection to the universe led me to start writing my observations while continuing to study science, history, philosophy, and spirituality. In my early forties, I embraced Christianity and began to study the Bible, which provided me with profound insights and clarity, answering many of my long-standing questions.

Five years ago, driven by a desire to serve my patients better and reach a broader audience, I began writing this motivational and practical self-improvement book. I aim to share my perspectives and extend the benefits beyond my medical practice to anyone open to exploring.

My lifelong admiration and deep respect for nature also found expression in photography, first as a hobby and later as a professional pursuit. My landscape and seascape art is showcased in local galleries, and I have published two coffee table books.

—*Razvan Balotescu, MD*

Acknowledgments

I would particularly like to thank Winston Parker, my spiritual teacher, for his unwavering guidance and support, and Nicolae Trif, my inspiring and passionate middle school math teacher, whose enthusiasm ignited my love for learning. To my editors, Michelle Williamson, Tessa Hall, Emily Carmain, and Don Weise, who endured listening to me and tirelessly read and restructured all my disorganized writings—your patience and expertise have been invaluable. Special thanks to Dragos Alexandrescu for keeping me updated on world events and broadening my perspective. To the many patients who have taught and inspired me in my quest for better care—your insights, stories, and experiences have profoundly shaped this journey. Last but not least, I thank my wife, Petronella, and my parents, Maria and Ion, for their continuous tolerance, encouragement, and support.

Introduction

Comfort without challenge will kill you.

Imagine you're riding a mountain bike with its sturdy frame and the wide, knobby tires that grip the ground on rocky trails. But today, somehow, you find yourself on a smooth, sleek racing track. As you start pedaling, the tires, meant for rugged terrain, struggle on unfamiliar ground, and the suspension, designed for bumps and jumps, remains inactive. It's like a trail runner attempting to sprint in high heels. Your progress is slow and becomes destructive.

Why? There is an obvious mismatch between the bike's design and its function, purpose, and use.

You and I have a similar problem, not as obvious but very damaging. It can cripple us, slowly but surely. Humanity never had this issue until recently, for the past few decades.

The new modern lifestyle poses a significant health threat. And I'm not talking about pollution, new chemicals, or other man-made harmful substances, which I will address later in the book. They also add to our health problems, but this is worse.

The issue is that we live in a bubble that creates a mismatch between our design and our lifestyle. Our design refers to the way we, as a species, are made functional and structurally adapted to the way we have lived for many thousands of years, which, significantly, was mostly the same until recently.

With the help of technology, modern culture has created a toxic bubble that is engulfing us. This bubble, which consists of our environment—physical, social, psychological, and so on—disconnects us from who we are, from nature, and from our ancestors. It is the main reason we suffer from most chronic diseases. It hurts us far beyond the physical level.

How is this happening?

Let me illustrate. Do you agree that it is a lot easier to gain weight than to lose weight? The fact is, your body instincts think you're still a caveman, and you must still build reserves and fatten, regardless of how much you are eating or how much food you have. Our genes and inner body intelligence are designed, and work based on how our ancestors lived for many thousands of years when food was scarce. The genes and instincts don't know we live in a new technological era; they don't understand modern life, where food is readily available and not moving doesn't kill you anymore.

We are pre-designed by our ancestors' way of life, how they lived for many thousands of years. Our lifestyle changed a lot after the Industrial Revolution a couple of hundred years ago. But it changed significantly faster in the past few decades due to the rapid and radical changes of modern technology.

Some may argue that it is no big deal, as we have always adapted to the changes. There are two problems with this view.

One, adaptation takes a long time, is a burden, and costs us all a lot of suffering. Look at what happened when we changed our lifestyle from hunter-gatherers to farmers. According to the evidence of skeletons from those periods in our evolution, the average human body shrank three inches in height and developed multiple chronic inflammatory conditions. This is primarily due to a significant increase in the amount of carbs we started to consume on a regular basis by introducing agricultural products—even if the amount of carbs we had then was far less than we have today.

Second, changes are now happening continuously, too rapidly and too radically, and we will not have time to adapt. After over 5,000 years, we are still not fully adapted to the farmer's diet. Many people still have intolerance to gluten and other grains.

The change from the farmer lifestyle, which lasted many thousands of years, to modern times is at least as abrupt and aggressive as it was from the caveman to the farmer.

Comfort without challenge will hurt or even kill you.

Until recently, we did not have modern technology conveniences, so life was harsh and a lot more challenging. Challenges not only helped us evolve but also made us thrive and be successful. They made us stronger.

However, lately, thanks to advancing technology and cultural shifts, we have been avoiding these challenges. We live in a culture that seeks comfort and pleasure almost exclusively, and as a result, we become weaker and unhealthy. In my community, the decrease in prices and the increase in the availability of electric bikes and scooters in the past few years made most people switch from manual bikes to them.

Think about this question: How healthy or rather unhealthy are you? In fact, how do you measure health? Modern culture makes us believe that being healthy means having no detectable disease, having normal medical tests, and feeling fine. After twenty-five years of internal medicine practice as a primary care physician, following thousands of patients every year, I can confidently say that is far from the truth.

I remember a new patient in his early sixties who had been swimming six days a week, forty to fifty minutes, for the past ten years. Over that time, he had unremarkable, normal blood tests and no physical complaints except some minor sleeping issues. I was surprised that one day he developed acute chest pain, and he ended up having open heart surgery with triple bypass. He did not have any obvious risk factors, like a family history of early coronary artery disease, smoking, or alcohol abuse.

So, what happened? How could this man develop heart disease despite regular swimming? I asked him how he swam and whether he was pushing at all. He said he took his time with no real effort, more like a stroll. So that is the problem: he was not uncomfortable at all while swimming. It was just a relaxing pace rather than a workout. This is precisely why swimming was not protecting him; there was no challenge, no hardship. He was not doing any other type of demanding activity either. He also admitted he went through long periods of high stress in the past but nothing in the last five years since he retired.

Some challenges and conflicts are an unavoidable but necessary part of life. Without them, we could not grow, adapt, and become stronger. They produce stress and suffering necessary for our adaptation, survival, and thriving. An example is when a new sibling is born, and the older child then must share the parents' attention and other benefits.

As Roman poet Persius wrote long ago, "He conquers who endures."

There is much unavoidable pain; nature is not fair. Accidents, death, genetic traits and defects, and natural disasters are part of this. They are beyond our control, and there is little we can do to prevent them. But we can improve the way we handle them.

Yet there is also a lot of avoidable, unnecessary suffering. This kind of suffering is only found in humans; animals do not have this problem. It is due to our conscious mind, which greatly expands our freedom of choice. The uneducated conscious mind, in its freedom, mistakenly chooses to ignore our design and our ancient wisdom and abuse what it likes, often without limits. It affects us and the people we are connected with. We abuse because we can. Animals would do that too, but they do not have the possibility unless we enable them. I am thinking here about the little fat dog of our obese neighbor. We are all looking for gratification, we are pleasure-seeking beings.

You may ask, unnecessary for what? The brief answer is for our well-being and for increasing our ability to pursue and fulfill creative, higher purposes.

If much of our suffering—whether physical, mental, or spiritual—is unnecessary and self-induced, how can we reduce and minimize this?

First, we need to understand human nature and nature in general. Self-induced suffering is ancient and due to destructive human nature, as this book explains. And then there is the toxic bubble of modern times.

The burden of adapting to novel, unnatural challenges.

The modern, harmful, way of life, in a nutshell, consists of two important facts. One is the mismatch presented above between our human design and our lifestyle, as the latter has changed dramatically. The other fact is how modern times amplify our basic, destructive human nature through a significantly expanded number of options, because of technological advances.

The solution is easy: recognize and respect our design—our body and mind's predetermined characteristics and functions and their purposes—and change our lifestyle so it matches the design.

Technology has brought us a lot of comfort, which is supposed to protect us from most of the pain and discomfort we have had for centuries. Today, we are more protected from severe injuries, trauma, and acute disease, but new forms of chronic pain and suffering unknown in the past are exploding.

The bubble we've created isolates us and keeps us away from natural challenges that used to make us stronger and better. This bubble gives us a false sense of well-being. It results from today's culture, which is abandoning previous wisdom and following new ideas fueled by our manipulated primitive drives instead. For example, replacing family as the pillar of our society with individual priorities has led to increased divorce rates, single-parent children, and fewer children per family, also resulting in significant population aging with a risk of extinction.

On a positive note, the challenges in sports and fair competitions are now part of our culture. They match our design and have important positive effects. But they're not persistent and widespread enough for most of us to prevent or fix this destructive bubble effect.

The old fundamental problem, the basic destructive human nature, needs spirituality to improve it and to reduce the suffering it causes.

This book offers a blueprint to unveil tools that will equip you to handle conflicts between biological, physical, and cultural forces. Much of the foundational knowledge is rooted in ancient wisdom that I have reformulated to fit today's world. It will help you better understand how you work and how to be healthy.

In these chapters, I share my secrets for applying this old wisdom, merged with modern science, to achieve ultimate health, less suffering, and discover your true purpose.

When armed with greater purposes, it is much easier to fight against our mind-twisted primitive nature, evolve into our spiritual nature, and thrive in wisdom.

A quick note on human and nature's intelligence.

There are at least two distinct types of intelligence. The first is the intelligence of nature, which made all of life possible; we could call it nature's mind. The second is the type that makes us aware and gives us the conscious mind—the human mind.

We humans are partially animals. Our very design causes us, to a large extent, to be driven by primitive instincts and drives. Yet, while an animal's instincts follow nature's intelligence and align with the ultimate purpose of its creation, our *conscious mind often manipulates our drives*. It can push us in a destructive direction. Conscious minds frequently disconnect us from nature's intelligence.

What motivates individuals to engage in unhealthy behaviors?

Our conscious mind can misuse and twist our basic instincts—primitive drives—which initially existed to protect us and ensure our survival.

Humans have a plethora of choices available to them daily. The capability to make these choices comes from the conscious mind. Consequently, decisions, behaviors, actions, and the adverse outcomes they often lead to are responsible for much human hardship and self-destruction.

On a positive note, a conscious mind is the reason humanity evolved so much, and it can be very constructive. However, people also engage in detrimental activities because they have the capacity to create diverse but often harmful new options, usually neglecting the consequences or failing to recognize their damaging nature.

In other words, since your conscious mind is not subject to the protective nature's intelligence and natural selection, you become vulnerable.

Let me give you an example to help illustrate this. The American food industry, which has changed over the past century, is not developed to help you reap optimum health. Instead, it's the opposite. Through its massive variety of mostly unhealthy processed products, it can easily tempt you—or anybody—toward abuse, resulting in poor health, obesity, depression, and so on.

The sad thing is that all too often, we are not aware of the mental flaw that makes us so vulnerable.

That, my friend, ends here.

You will come away from this book with the following questions answered:

- *What specific lifestyle aspects do not fit our natural design, damaging our health, and how can I correct them?*
- *Why are there so many diets, and still, none is right for everyone? Why is eating according to our design the only correct way to get healthy and stay healthy?*
- *What is the original, often hidden trigger in making many important decisions or actions?*
- *How can I replace my destructive habits with healthy ones?*
- *What higher purposes should I strive to achieve to live a fulfilling life?*

The book is structured so that each chapter can be read individually.

The first two chapters address the connections between our lifestyle, health, and genetic-biological design with the explosion of chronic diseases.

Chapters 3 to 10 present and help you implement the most important eight lifestyle habits that can improve your health and well-being.

Chapter 11 introduces you to the concept of measuring and trading the discomfort required to implement healthy habits successfully.

Chapter 12 addresses our human nature flaws that contribute to developing harmful bad habits and unnecessary suffering.

Chapter 13 gives a broad medical perspective on the explosion of chronic diseases, why they occur, and how to handle them by addressing the root causes rather than the symptoms. It also discusses how our new toxic culture influences conventional medicine.

Chapters 14 to 16 dive into how nature works inside and around us so we can achieve complete health and how to use this knowledge to find meanings and purposes.

Chapter 17 addresses human nature's broader harmful social consequences and how to reduce its destructive effects.

You don't need to be your own worst enemy any longer. You will become equipped with applications and practices to make life-transforming changes.

Are you ready to break the toxic bubble?

Let's begin this journey by discovering how to improve your health by rematching your lifestyle with your natural inherited design.

Chapter 1

The Power of Inherited Design

We are pre-designed by our ancestors' way of life.

Do you want to achieve optimal health and excel in all avenues of life? If so, it's vital to learn and respect your inherited design. The truth is, despite our self-destructive nature, our evolution is assured by design. Our predecessors struggled to survive, and their success created an important inherited mechanism. We have been gifted with a powerful tool that has made civilization survive and prosper. Thanks to nature's intelligence, we are designed to respond and change according to demands, and we can inherit and transmit the gains achieved. This inherited feature, known as *adaptation*, is alive and well in our genes and remains essential for evolution and survival.

The reality is this: we are pre-designed by our ancestors' way of life, and we are born adapted to their lifestyle. Whatever we do—whether we implement a new diet or start a new activity—it is important that we first consider our design. Why is it important for us to consider how our ancestors lived? If our diet or activities do *not* fit our design, there is a good chance we could either harm ourselves or have difficulty coping. We must respect the genes that encode our design because they are a dominant part of who we are and how we are structured. Using a tool for a purpose that goes against its structure is never a wise idea. Have you tried to open a beer bottle with your teeth?

Don't do it. It doesn't feel good and can damage your teeth and even your jaw.

Adaptation to new undertakings used outside our design should be avoided and only used if we find ourselves out of options. In other words, we should use our bodies for their intended purpose whenever possible rather than trying to adapt to do something the human body was not designed for. Unfortunately, in the new modern bubble, we are surrounded by completely new challenges that our ancestors historically had never seen.

As humans, it is part of our design to survive. This fight for survival was constantly on the minds of our ancestors. For thousands of years, life was harsh, and food was difficult for them to find. They did not have the options that we have today, so they ate much less and lived a more active lifestyle.

Many other important aspects of our daily lives have remained unchanged since the beginning of human civilization until just a few generations ago. From the way we sit to the way we sleep, from the way we move to the way we relate, most of our routines and daily activities have changed radically. As I mentioned, most of these changes are detrimental to our health.

So, first, how have essential aspects of life, such as eating, moving, and mind activities, changed in modern times? And how do they challenge our design? Later, I review some other routine contemporary lifestyle aspects, which are also responsible for many of our modern chronic health problems.

Eating and the propensity for gaining weight.

I explained above why gaining weight is a lot easier than losing it. The answer lies in our *design*.

Caveman's genes still dominate us. Our hunger today is still powerful, driven by a survival instinct. Herbivores like horses and deer, in contrast, never gain weight, regardless of how much grass they eat. Their hunger is less intense than ours. There will always be more for the next day, as long as the fields remain green, so they don't need to overeat.

A large part of the dietary problems we have in America and other countries worldwide is that our eating patterns do not match our inherited genetic design. Up until the Industrial Revolution began 200 to 300 years ago, it would have been a privilege for our ancestors to have enjoyed even a single full meal each day. We are not designed to consume three meals and several snacks throughout the day.

As ancient wisdom and modern science prove, eating less food—and less frequently—is far better for our health. A twenty-four-hour or more fasting habit would mimic how our ancestors lived. It explains why intermittent fasting works so well. The health benefits of intermittent fasting are scientifically proven, and prolonged fasting was also used in ancient wisdom to promote physical and mental healing.

Since we could domesticate animals and grow food, we have changed some. Our resources were ever present, so we do not need to eat large meals anymore. We are genetically a mix of a few million years of living a hunter's lifestyle and a few thousand years of living a farmer's lifestyle. The changes we have made in the past fifty to one hundred years are too recent to make a significant difference, as it takes longer to adapt completely. Therefore, these changes are mostly an aggression toward our well-being.

The transition from a hunter-gatherer lifestyle to a more sedentary farming lifestyle, known as the Neolithic Revolution, led to a decline in overall health for our ancestors, at least initially.

This change happened because as societies began to rely more heavily on agriculture, they started eating a diet that was much higher in carbohydrates. This favored bacteria over-growth and radically changed our intestinal and respiratory flora. The increased consumption of carbohydrates also led to an increase in dental issues like cavities, which is obviously observed when we compare their skeletons and dentitions.

The nature of exercise.

Our ancestors led a very active lifestyle, which designed our body. Because of this, we, too, need to exercise regularly, which is crucial to maintaining good health today.

Let's consider what their daily activity looked like. They typically moved in random intervals with a variable pace as they hunted, gathered, or traveled on an inconsistent and diverse landscape, like the trails in the woods. This explains why interval training achieves optimum results compared to an exercise that involves a continuous pace. Even runners who train for a marathon use an interval training method, like moving with variable speed, because of its efficacy and since it is scientifically proven. This mimics our ancestors' way of moving. There is nothing in nature that is unvarying.

For example—if we run on a concrete, flat, straight path, or a treadmill at a consistent pace and for prolonged periods, we are at risk of injuries. The repetitive impact was uncommon for our ancestors and can become destructive for the joints that receive the most impact.

You may have experienced this yourself. Have you ever tried to run barefoot? This tends to be more natural for humans than wearing shoes. Running as though barefoot—or wearing near-barefoot shoes—is more protective of our joints since humans have done this for so long.

Here's what this looks like when performed accurately: The person runs with small steps, lands on the front foot with the knee bent, and avoids landing on the heels with straight legs.

For runners who train incorrectly, however, changing to the proper method that fits our design will need to occur progressively, as our foot muscles are weak and not adapted to take over most of the impact, as it happens when we start running barefoot or wearing near-barefoot shoes. Abrupt changes can become too aggressive and may even result in injuries.

Practically, if we run on concrete, we should run like we are barefoot but wearing thick, soft-sole shoes that reduce the mechanical stress and mimic the impact with grass and dirt.

The continuous increase in our pace of life significantly affects our mind.

Have you ever gone hiking or backpacking in the mountains for a few days straight, completely unplugged from electronics, the Internet, and phone signals? It's an experience that really slows things down and changes your perspective.

Before the days of modern technology, this was pretty much how people lived most of their lives. I remember one time when I was hiking in Patagonia, and after about three days, the silence became almost overwhelming. I started mentally playing my favorite songs just to fill the void. But after a few more days, I actually started to enjoy the peace and quiet.

Coming back to civilization was a shock. The noise and constant visual stimulation of the city felt like an assault on the senses. It took me a couple of days to get used to it again. But even then, I found myself missing the simplicity and tranquility of those days in the mountains.

Our modern physical lifestyle is more sedentary, but our mental pace has drastically increased. This has mostly occurred in the past twenty years or so—specifically once personal computers and smartphones were invented. We constantly multitask, are overstimulated, and our focus is often thrown in multiple directions. Yet this accelerated, high-speed pace of life is not healthy.

It's particularly unhealthy for young children. The young among us are significantly affected. How do I know this? Because of the increased incidence of attention deficit disorder (ADD), insomnia, and anxiety.

Nearly fifty percent of all teenagers have been prescribed ADD medication, even though statistically, only five to ten percent of the population is expected to develop the disorder as the result of a genetic predisposition.

A large study of five-year-olds published in the Canadian journal *BMC Public Health* compared the attention spans of kids who watched TV less than thirty minutes per day with those who spent more than two hours before a screen. The results were dramatic: The children who gazed the longest had 7.7 times more of a chance of meeting the criteria for an ADHD diagnosis.

Most of us have experienced the side effects of trying to keep up with our high-speed, fast-paced lifestyle. It is often associated with elevated levels of stress hormones like adrenaline and cortisol. It's no wonder there has been an increase in health issues such as ADD, anxiety, insomnia, fatigue, headaches, and depression in the past ten years! Sadly, the long-term effects are even life-threatening and include an increased incidence of cardiovascular diseases such as heart attacks, strokes, and cancer.

Living according to our design: more illustrations.

Let's put into practice more habits that our ancestors developed in all areas of life. Modern technology should facilitate rather than obstruct these applications.

Here are examples of some of the practices we should continue or restart from our ancestor's way of life:

Eat in season and from local sources of food, This should be your "diet."

As a newcomer to the United States thirty years ago, I was struck by the sight of watermelons being sold in grocery stores during the winter season. Coming from Romania, I was used to a lifestyle that revolved around seasonal produce. We only had access to fruits and vegetables that were in season, and we never mixed produce from different seasons in the same meal. For example, berries were only available in May and June, cherries in June and July, watermelons in August, and apples and grapes in September and October. Each season brought with it a unique set of fruits and vegetables that we eagerly looked forward to enjoying. I believe that a return to this seasonal way of living would not only benefit our health and well-being but also help support local farmers and promote sustainable agriculture.

Eating in season implies a reduced diversity of foods. This has a positive effect on our health. Humanity, for many thousands of years until a few generations ago, consumed the same kind of whole food and drink, limited to what was available through local farming for each season. For example, in the cold seasons, October to March, we were mostly carnivores, as there were no fresh fruits or vegetables available. There was no technology to produce and preserve the foods the way the food industry is extensively doing now. In fact, vegetables were available only for a few weeks in the spring and fruits for a few weeks in the summer and fall. We extended their availability by fermentation, for example, by making sauerkraut or by drying them, as in the case of dried fruits. After the Industrial Revolution, the food industry changed dramatically, particularly in the past few decades.

Ideally, local and in-season should be with respect to your ancestors' geographic location. For example, if you have ancestors primarily from northern Europe, then the food you eat should be mostly what was available in that region in each season for thousands of years.

This approach will enable us to enjoy fresh, unprocessed food while reducing our reliance on various food enhancements and manipulations necessary when food cannot be consumed immediately due to storage and transportation requirements. It also helps improve our digestion and metabolism efficiency. Consuming foods from four seasons and five continents in the same meal, as we so often do now, is overwhelming for our body's food processing mechanisms.

There are a few books that can provide detailed, specific information on how to eat and live locally and seasonally, like the popular and successful "It Starts with Food/The Whole30" series by Melissa and Dallas Hartwig.

We should minimize foods affected by genetic modifications, pesticides, and other unnatural human interventions. Many farms today are returning to the old ways of producing food. Advances in technology could make it much more manageable without interfering with the quality of the produce.

We should increase our consumption of wild fish and pasture-raised, locally grown, hormone- and antibiotic-free chickens and their eggs. Before the establishment of large farms in the early nineteenth century, red meat was not readily available, and most people couldn't afford to own a lot of livestock. Consuming wild game regularly is much better, but it is rarely possible today. Aside from the contamination from modern pollution, wild fish is the closest to but even better than wild game.

We should raise our animals and birds on pastures and outdoors and feed them like we always did, straight from the land.

The current conditions in large-scale industrial farms are disheartening; The animals are often abused, inoculated with growth hormones and antibiotics, and fed low-quality food. Their diet quality can impact our health as they become what they eat. We should avoid consuming them if we can. In large industrial farms, cage-raised chickens are one of the most abused and harmful to our health. They are, unfortunately, the most consumed, ubiquitously present in all grocery stores, fast food chains, and restaurants.

Go to bed or slow down early, soon after it gets dark, and wake up with the sunlight.

This is how our ancestors lived for thousands of years. Doing so would improve sleep quality, the next day's energy, and the retention of information assimilated the previous day. It can also relieve depression. Chapter 9 addresses modern sleep issues in more detail.

Expose yourself to sunlight early and late in the day to develop a protective suntan.

Sunlight is safe during the first and last hours of the day when there are low levels of damaging UV light.

Each of us should spend time or play outdoors as much as possible, surrounding ourselves with the natural elements found in the ground, the plants, and the animals. (Sadly, nowadays, in our environment, there are many new artificial chemicals—either man-made or modified—that may be harmful to our health.)

Add minerals to the drinking water.

Our ancestors used to drink "live" water straight from the ground, from wells or springs. This water was moving water, rich in minerals, microorganisms, and micronutrients. Today, most commercial water from grocery stores or taps is dead. Our bottled water, even the most expensive, has no taste, no microorganisms, no or low mineral content, and it's completely static. We must filter our water since it is contaminated. Unfortunately, this process also removes the good, important components in the water. What are the roles of nonpathogenic organisms usually found in the well and spring water? How much are we affected by their absence? Often, chlorine or fluoride is added to the water.

Just like the thirteen essential vitamins, there are over sixty essential minerals the body needs to function properly. We need them for proper immunity, hormone production, brain function, and many other purposes. Deficiency in minerals often leads to multiple chronic medical conditions, like osteoporosis, hypothyroidism, diabetes, cardiac arrhythmias, anemia, immune deficiencies and so on. Drinking water containing minerals may also reduce the craving for other drinks and foods, particularly foods rich in salt, many of which are unhealthy snacks. The best source of minerals for drinking water comes from Celtic or Himalayan salt put in a solution as they are purer and have a higher number of minerals. There are a few commercially available brands.

Fruits, vegetables, and most other crops are also lower in minerals than they used to be. This is because the soil has been depleted of minerals. As in modern, large-scale agriculture, there is little to no fertilization by recycling the wasted food or using animal manure.

Carbonated drinks, so common nowadays, are new to the body. These can be harmful because of their high carbon dioxide content, which can form unhealthy combinations with our body's minerals, particularly if consumed in high amounts. They can commonly produce joint inflammation and osteoporosis.

Drinking regular water that is low in minerals, especially if we do it fast and in a high amount, will lead to body waste of minerals in the urine along with increased diuresis, as the body doesn't like the sudden dilution of the blood. This also contributes to the significant increase in osteoporosis incidents in the general population.

End your showers with cold water. Go further and practice cold plunges on a regular basis.

Incorporating cold water into your shower routine provides several benefits, particularly when contrasted with hot water. Having only warm or hot showers without exposure to cold water is also novel and undesirable for our design. Remember, we never had warm water and plumbing until 100-plus years ago. We mostly washed with freezing cold water, especially in the colder seasons. There are numerous advantages of using cold water and contrast temperatures, and you can find a detailed explanation in the contrast temperatures chapter, Chapter 4.

Sit straight on a hard chair without back or arm support.

Alternate between your regular soft cushioned desk chair and an old-fashioned simple chair without support and with minimal cushion. Pay attention to your posture. Sit and walk like you're carrying a plate on top of your head. I have seen hundreds and probably thousands of back X-rays and MRIs in my twenty-five years of practice. The majority of adults, even those in their thirties and forties, have multiple spine disk damage, bone spurs, and other chronic degenerative conditions. Many are asymptomatic till one day when, unsurprisingly, the acute followed by chronic back pain starts. I blame it mainly on how we sit and weaken core muscles. This is mainly due to spending hundreds of hours a month in an improperly crouched, "comfortable" position in soft chairs with cushioned backrests. No backrest, the way we always used to sit until a few generations ago, is better than the improper modern ones with a backrest (the vast majority) and probably better even than the ergonomic backrest ones.

Be careful with machines and other guided exercise devices when working out at the gym.

It's optimal for our joints and muscles to use free weights and free movements instead of machines. For most of us, the best way to strengthen our bodies is to practice functional movements using mostly our body weight or just low weights.

Take frequent, short breaks from looking at nearby screens.

Instead, we should direct our gaze toward the outdoors through a window. Our ancestors spent only a little time indoors or looking at close-up objects. Continuous and persistent close-up viewing can lead to eye strain, muscle tension, and headaches.

Have newborns delivered naturally as we always did until very recently.

This involves several factors and steps, one of which is delaying the clamping and cutting of the umbilical cord after delivery. It is known as "delayed cord clamping." The benefits for the baby are significant and risk-free. They include increased blood volume, higher hemoglobin levels, improved iron stores, better transition to the outside world with respiratory and neurodevelopmental advantages, and improved stem cell availability. More early skin-to-skin contact between the mother and baby provides better temperature regulation for the baby, increased breastfeeding success, and the establishment of the mother's natural flora in the baby's digestive system.

Women couldn't have cesarean sections until recent times. It is advisable to minimize the use of C-sections whenever possible. C-section deliveries have been associated with a lack of healthy flora in newborns, which can contribute to developing chronic medical conditions later in life, such as obesity and chronic allergies.

Natural vaginal birth provides protective bacterial flora from the mother to the newborns, which is crucial for their later healthy development. This is why in some northern European countries, hospitals routinely apply swabs from the mother's vagina to the C-section newborn's mouth. Sadly, there is very little research and interest in this important area of medicine.

We pay a high price for not respecting our biological design. The modern culture encourages having fewer babies, which has led to an increasing incidence of breast and other cancers. Women who have multiple pregnancies and breastfeed experience a significant reduction in the risk of breast, ovarian, and endometrial cancers, as well as multiple sclerosis, rheumatoid arthritis, and other autoimmune diseases.

Avoid living in isolation.

Unfortunately, this way of life is common nowadays, thanks to advanced technology. It wasn't always this way, though. For thousands of years, it was common for people to grow up in large families. Also, people could only isolate for a short time; for survival, they had to work together to find food or stay protected from danger.

Children have always played in groups. Unfortunately, in the past decades, this has been happening less and less, particularly in developed countries. Early in life, playing and interacting with other children is important for the development of personality, individuality, and character. Virtual interactions through digital screens, social media, and other applications do not provide the same benefits, and they can be harmful.

Many studies, like the ones from the Meta-Analysis by Holt-Lunstad et al. (2010), show that if we hope to live a long, quality life, we must surround ourselves with people. This is a contributing factor to attaining a fulfilling life. It's vital for our health that we establish good relationships with those around us—relationships rooted in love and deep care for the other person's well-being.

Adding a pet to the family, especially a dog, is another positive factor in obtaining this quality of life. Studies have also proven that having a pet helps us live longer—probably because good relationships improve our well-being. The increased number of pets in recent generations is a positive factor, which probably helps to compensate for the reduced interaction with our peers nowadays.

Incorporate physical stimulation of different body parts into your daily routine.

Living in modern times is like living in a bubble, "protected" from many exposures to natural stimulations of our senses. These come in many forms, including physical and mechanical.

Traditional Chinese medicine practices, like chi-gong, often involve self-tapping, squeezing, and rubbing various body areas. For example, one method of tooth stimulation is intense and regular teeth clenching as part of overall body stimulation exercises. Our modern diet does not provide the benefits of this action, such as increased blood flow and strengthening the teeth roots and gums. Our ancestors consumed foods with a greater abundance of plant roots and meat off the bones, necessitating more chewing and biting.

By integrating these practices into our daily routine, we can reap the benefits of stimulating different body systems and promoting overall well-being.

The list of health improvements and positive habits we can and should practice continues.

The life span question.

One may wonder why our ancestors' life span was much shorter than ours. That is mainly because they could not treat life-threatening conditions as well as we do today, like acute injuries and acute diseases such as infections or bleeding. We can even see how we used to live if we look at those who live in remote areas in the Amazon Forest, Africa, or Australia. These people live in tribes and have ways of life similar to those of our ancestors. The incidence of chronic diseases in these populations is much lower, and there are low rates of coronary artery disease, degenerative, autoimmune, vascular disease, and cancer in these areas. We live longer in the civilized world mostly because we have immediate access to emergency medicine and treatments for acute illnesses such as infections, trauma, allergic reactions, and so forth.

Technology protects us. This is especially true when we consider that good hygiene, air conditioning, clean sanitation, and immediate access to health care are almost universal in Western societies.

The positive addition of our ancestors' wisdom and practice.

We can benefit a great deal from learning about treasures found in ancient wisdom. Following hundreds of years of intelligent observation, this ancient wisdom added new influences on our design.

For example, meditation, yoga, chi-gong, and tai chi respect our body and mind's design. These types of practices added new movements and postures that were copied from the behavior of animals and birds. All these techniques and others like acupuncture, massage, and physical therapies have one important thing in common. They demand and stimulate our body; they challenge us, so the body naturally responds by adapting to them. This results in faster healing, increased strength, and better health. They were carefully created, implemented, and adjusted to our design to prevent injuries. And, of course, the test of time subjected them to natural selection and eliminated the unsuccessful ones.

Many traditional Asian texts detail food combinations and their effects on the body. The Chinese have a science dedicated to the effect of individual foods on our health, as well as the compatibility and effects of different food combinations—all this while respecting the local and in-season concept. For example they have specific recommendations for certain foods to be consumed at certain times of the day.

Another method from ancient wisdom that can improve our lives involves the way we eat. When our ancestors advanced, and food became less scarce, they no longer needed to eat fast to ensure they consumed enough food to survive until their next meal could be found. So even though our survival instinct pushes us to eat fast and large portions, it is best for our health and digestion to slow down when we eat and chew our food well. This is especially true since we often eat more diverse foods within the same meal.

Most spiritual texts and traditions, regardless of their religion or geographic location, promote specific eating habits. These practices often involve restrictions on certain foods for certain periods, including partial or complete fasting. The purpose behind these restrictive dietary guidelines is to promote spiritual and physical strengthening while avoiding overindulgence, even though the food was scarce for most. Despite being a part of our ancestors' lives, these customs have been largely erased today by modern culture when we would need them the most, as food abuse and abundance have reached unprecedented harmful levels.

Want to obtain optimal health? Let's adopt these practices from our ancestors.

Why do you think it's healthier for us to eat fish rather than beef or chicken? And why are omega-3 oils better for us than other animal fats? The reason is that fish and its omega-3-rich fats are older and have been more frequently consumed by humans. Since we are designed to adapt to survival and evolution demands, we adapted to fish better because we ate fish so frequently and in high amounts for the most extended period. Our bodies have processed fish longer. Therefore, its digestion and processing are smoother and occur faster than when we eat other types of meat.

The longer a type of food has been present in the human diet, and the more of it has been eaten, the better the human body adapted to it. Thus, it became more valuable and healthier for us over time. But it takes many hundreds and thousands of years to be complete.

It's interesting to see how, throughout history, most populations developed around bodies of water. Do you know why? Humans were drawn to water since it is a rich and easy food source. Therefore, they ate fish so much and for so many centuries. This created the "beaten paths" for our bodies to process and metabolize the proteins and fats from the fish.

As cavemen and hunters, we ate more wild game and wild plants but involuntarily fasted more than we do today. Later, the farmers ate less meat and more vegetables and fasted less.

Red meat, like beef and pork, was not readily available, even for farmers. They would not kill their own animals that often, so hunting was more likely to provide red meat. Eggs and chickens were more readily available, so they were consumed more often than red meat.

There is also a significant difference among different regions, continents, and periods concerning access to red meat, plants, and other foods. The newest genetic testing can help us better determine our ancestors' genetic characteristics. This information can then be used to determine their lifestyle and diet. We must consider it to learn how to adjust our diet and eating habits.

So, what is the bottom line that we must grasp? To put it simply, fish is healthier than meat and even vegetables. We can also see great results when we fast—and even better results if we mix fasting with a paleo-caveman diet.

A good rule of thumb is this: *The more recently a food has been introduced into our diet, the more difficult it is for us to process and metabolize.* If the food is newer, we will likely have incomplete processing and waste. This then leads to inflammation, which, of course, becomes a burden for our bodies. Many people have side effects from eating grains, particularly wheat and gluten. Besides being introduced later in our regular diet, they are further genetically modified and processed. Look at the health problems discovered in the skeletons of the first generations of farmers as they transitioned from hunter and gatherer lifestyle.

Taking supplements is not the same as getting the same micronutrients from food—and does not result in the same health benefits. It's far more ideal for us to consume the vitamins from our foods. Vitamin C or B12, for example, gets naturally absorbed in the digestive tract from the food we eat—not so much from supplements, though.

Not all carbs are the same.

Honey, probably the oldest high-carb food, is one of the fastest metabolized carbohydrates, as the blood sugar level after eating honey decreases quickly in minutes. The more processed a carbohydrate is, the less our receptors will recognize it. This can then cause the highly processed carbohydrate to remain in the blood longer, and *that* can cause damage to our blood vessels.

Honey has created a "beaten path" in our bodies. Our ancestors ate honey for thousands of years, so our bodies tend to recognize and process it quickly.

The newer carbohydrates have different (new and unfamiliar) structures that are neither recognized nor processed as easily. These newer carbohydrates do not have a fast, smooth metabolic path. So, not only do these carbohydrates linger in the blood longer before they become metabolized, but they are also not completely utilized. This creates waste that requires inflammatory cells for its removal.

If we eat different products containing processed carbohydrates—for example, high fructose corn syrup, evaporated canned sugar, Splenda, aspartame, and other substitutes—our blood sugar levels will stay elevated for several hours upon their consumption.

The waste becomes a burden and increases inflammation in the body. This inflammation can trigger, exacerbate, or even produce chronic inflammatory diseases, such as psoriasis, inflammatory bowel disease, thyroid disease, diabetes, chronic sinus allergies, and asthma.

Many diets result in some degree of success simply because they remove unhealthy eating habits and processed carbohydrates. It is important to remember, though, that the closer a diet is to matching our genetic, inherited design, the higher the chances we have of receiving sustained healthy results with that diet. Why are there so many success stories from people using even opposite diets, like carnivore versus vegetarian diets? Besides the important thing—that we remove junk food—we eat more consciously and usually disciplined and in lower amounts. Also, we adapt more easily to a particular diet as there is more consistency over time.

This is also because, as I discussed earlier, the human body is designed to eat less diverse foods, and we have always eaten locally and in season, which limits diversity. This makes digestion and metabolism more efficient, and we develop an intestinal flora that is more specialized and more efficient. Eating in one meal or in one day foods that come from a wide variety of sources, different seasons, and different geographic locations ... it's too much for our body, and it's definitely not according to our design and our ancestors' way of life.

In my neighborhood, daily walks often reveal stories not spoken but seen. A tale of two Labradors perfectly encapsulates this.

The first Labrador, a five-year-old chocolate-coated fellow, has a broad, square body that struggles with every step. His owner, a kind-hearted woman with similar health challenges, often shares her own meals with him—mostly leftovers from her table, which are far from tailored to a dog's nutritional needs. Their shared eating habits form a bond, but unfortunately, it's one that compromises their health rather than enhances it.

Just down the street lives another Labrador, nine years old but with an unmistakable zest for life. His owner, a meticulous woman, selects only the finest cuts of meat for him, each piece carefully chosen from the local butcher's best. Her philosophy is simple: "Only the best for him." This Lab moves with the ease of a much younger dog, his coat glossy and his eyes bright with vitality.

If we can devote such care to feeding our pets well, why not extend the same consideration to ourselves? What if we treated our own bodies with the same respect and attentiveness that we often show our pets?

Imagine for a moment that you are the pet, reliant on someone who loves you dearly. Wouldn't you hope they chose the best, healthiest options for you?

The environmental impact on the body and genes, epigenetics.

The environmental factors that persisted for hundreds and thousands of years eventually became stronger and more dominant for the genetic adaptive response. They become imprinted and inherited in every generation; thus, they are difficult to change. But we are also genetically designed to adapt to temporary and less persistent demands. Then, once those demands stop, it takes almost as long for the genetic features to disappear as they did for them to appear.

Here is an experiment that illustrates this. A female mouse was exposed to an electric shock whenever she smelled a specific odor. She learned to run away when she smelled that odor. This mouse then became pregnant. Here's the interesting part: The baby mice were also exposed to that smell—without experiencing any associated electrical shock. Regardless, they, too, ran away.

Even when the offspring were separated from the mother at birth, the fear of the same smell was transmitted to the off-spring. This phenomenon is called *epigenetics*, and it is an essential mechanism for both survival and adaptation. (I want to clarify that, in this book, I use the terms "genetics" and "epigenetics" interchangeably.)

In the same way, political leanings and religious preferences are primarily inherited from our parents and grandparents.

Information is captured and transmitted through our genes. The purpose is to help offspring adapt quickly and in the best way they can.

Our ability to adapt, from a genetic perspective, is determined by the interplay between two sets of genes: the old, persistent genes that are dominant and the newer, temporary adaptive genes that have developed more recently as a response to newer environmental pressure.

On the other hand, our design is not just inherited. Because we adapted to our living conditions, we are partially formed by our experiences and personal history. Everyone has a unique gut flora that affects our response to what we eat. We also have unique weaknesses and strengths inherited from our parents and grandparents. Our blood type can also affect our response to food and the environment.

These complex factors influence our response to a particular diet or activity. We can only know how to respond by *experimenting* and *observing*. Genetic commercial tests are available today to help us determine how we process certain nutrients. These tests also analyze our gut bacteria. However, even though these tests may be helpful, they are not yet complete and accurate enough to deliver closer to one hundred percent accurate results.

Protective genes.

Life, naturally, inherently moves toward organization. There is a universal constructive force that makes this happen. I will describe it in depth in Chapter 14. This force also exists within our genes so we can grow up and reproduce. We must grow, reproduce, and protect our offspring until they can do the same. Harmful traits mostly appear and start to manifest once we are older, usually after age thirty. Essentially, each generation is protected from early bad gene expressions so we can live long enough to reproduce. These mechanisms protect us from disease gene expression. This is to ensure that our offspring are taken care of.

This explains why kids generally don't have many chronic diseases. It has to do with our genetic design. We were designed to protect and care for our offspring. To ensure that they survive and thrive. We are just beginning to understand these genes, called enhancer and silencer genes, and still know very little about them and how they regulate our gene expressions.

We wish our bad genes would be silenced until we're older than fifty or sixty, but this doesn't happen.

But there's a solution. We have the ability to influence the activation of certain genes by exposing our bodies to specific demanding conditions. Essentially, we can harness nature's wisdom to make our genes believe that we are in *survival mode*. Activities like intense exercise, fasting, or exposure to extreme temperatures (such as ice baths) signal to our genes that we are enduring challenges.

Genes cannot distinguish between deliberate challenges and actual threats. Historically, when our heart rates increased, when we went without food, or when we experienced discomfort from cold exposure, for example, our genes interpreted these signals as signs of danger, prompting a need for support and resilience. This is why certain "challenging" activities have been historically and scientifically shown to lower the risks of conditions like Alzheimer's, cardiovascular disease, and cancer. It's fascinating how having a clear purpose and striving towards it can put us in a state of survival mode, allowing us to achieve great things. I've always been amazed at how individuals in their eighties, who hold important functions and responsibilities, manage to perform so well and keep diseases at bay. It's a testament to the power of determination and having a clear sense of direction in life.

The opportunity for the recurring and complete renewal.

You may have thought that age and wear and tear are the leading causes of chronic health issues. But that's not true. They have almost nothing to do with age.

Almost one hundred percent of the body's cells are turned over within a given seven-to-ten-year period. We decompose and recompose.

Your brain, heart, bones, and even some scars are fully or partially recreated, all at different speeds. This process happens faster or slower for various types of tissues. The brain, bones, and nerve tissues regenerate slowest.

You are not the same person you were a decade ago. Almost every cell of your body has been renewed. How cool to think that we get a total makeover every seven to ten years!

Life is a cycle of renewal, but over time everything deteriorates. Constant renewal would make us think we can live forever, that nature wants us to live longer. But sadly, we renew everything—the chronic damage, the inflammation, even the bad genes. Our tendency toward destruction is renewed, too; it doesn't go away. It isn't natural for things to last forever.

The exciting news is that if we can change our habits, we can slow down the deterioration process. Suppose we persist in a new habit longer than the renewal period. In that case, we will renew differently because a persisting habit affects us on both mental and physical levels, all the way to the gene expressions involved in the renewal processes. This renewal could go either way—toward health or disease.

It all depends on the kind of habits we practice.

In summary:

We all encounter a modern, new issue: Our culture, lifestyle, and environment have changed radically, but human nature—physical, mental, and emotional—has not changed since the caveman era many thousands of years ago.

Our design is inherited and reflects the way humanity lived, which also has not changed much for many thousands of years till very recently. To change our design takes hundreds and thousands of years.

There is a significant mismatch between our modern lifestyle and our design. Our lifestyle had been the same until only a few generations ago.

This mismatch is the main cause of the modern explosion of chronic diseases. It creates damage beyond our physical health into our emotional, social, and spiritual health.

The only solution is to rematch our lifestyle with our design by changing our lifestyle, as our design cannot be changed significantly and fast enough—it takes many generations to do so.

These specific lifestyle changes, from how we move to how we eat and relate, could be easily recognized in our ancestors' lives, and reapplied nowadays with proven results for our health and well-being. In the next chapter, I will reveal how this rematch can be achieved and sustained successfully.

Chapter 2

The Power of Habits and Repetitive Demands

"Excellence is an art won by training and habituation: we do not act rightly because we have virtue or excellence, but we rather have these because we have acted rightly; 'these virtues are formed in man by his doing the actions'; we are what we repeatedly do. Excellence, then, is not an act but a habit."

—Will Durant, American writer, historian, and philosopher

Humans are habitual beings, and our habits have power. Most of our life is habitual, from daily habits like a morning alarm and cup of coffee to hourly habits like checking our phone for new messages or emails. In many ways, our habits both form and define us. We become attached to and dependent on our habits because they provide comfort, security, and joy—especially when immediate. In many cases, their long-term effect, however, might cause harm.

"Habit, if not resisted, soon becomes a necessity."

—St. Augustine

Some habits develop naturally as they satisfy daily needs. Others are imposed on us by our circumstances and environment—still others, we adopt voluntarily.

We are born with a genetically pre-designed brain map, but how we live will change the size and speed of our different "roads" and create new neuron connections, new "routes." When we repeatedly do something, we strengthen the neural connections involved in it. When we stop doing something, after a while, we weaken or even lose its corresponding connections.

Habits' functional maps inside of our brains are made of patterns of "beaten paths." These paths include high-speed neuronal connections. Here's a way to picture what happens: If a road or path is traveled repeatedly, it will get faster and broader (the road gets beaten down). Similarly, any repetitive, sustained neurological activity, in time, creates a faster, wider "path" of connection between involved neurons.

The more we use knowledge or participate in an activity, the faster and more proficient we become. This is the primary mechanism of learning, progressing, and perfecting.

Demanding by repetitive, persisting action is the key.

Habits are powerful. What makes them happen is not wishes or hopes but *daily demands*.

> *"We first make our habits; then our habits make us."*
> —John Dryden, influential English poet, playwright,
> and literary critic

Adaptation manifests in us from birth onward. It's the reason we can learn to ride a bike or drive a car. Anyone who does ten to twenty pushups twice daily for two weeks will develop visible, better definition in the arm and chest muscles. These are all good examples of adaptation.

We must take advantage of the body's almost unlimited potential to transform and adapt if we wish to change. Let's allow this to improve us. Here's the secret: We *can* change—but only if we wisely create our habits and develop self-discipline and perseverance. Then, our intelligent inherited genetic mechanisms will change us. Soon, we'll begin to adapt to the new demands and become stronger and healthier.

First, we need to align our will to a good, constructive principle or health concepts, and then we align our behavior and emotions to our will. Our actions, of course, will follow the direction of our will.

So, we only need to demand health from our body in order to receive it.

The process sounds too simple to be true. Of course, I'm not claiming that sustaining demand and discipline will be an easy process. Not necessarily. However, through habits and behavioral changes, we adapt, and accepting challenges becomes easier as we become accustomed to them.

"Natural forces within us are the true healers of disease."
—Hippocrates

The body has a huge capacity for self-healing that helps it survive, recover, and function after the various acute illnesses or injuries we experience. But when an injury is inflicted repetitively through unhealthy habits like smoking, eating fast foods, or drinking heavily, the body's self-healing mechanisms become overwhelmed, and we develop chronic illnesses.

Implementing a new habit.

Ready to adopt concepts that will help implement healthy new habits successfully?

1. Involve somebody else or pay for a class or personal trainer.

You don't have to face a new habit alone. Find an accountability partner, group, or trainer. According to several studies, you are much more likely to sustain a new habit if you involve others or if you're spending money to do it. It's even better if you can find a partner or group of like-minded people who are working toward the same goals, like qualifying and running a popular race. Recognize that it is crucial to work with people who support you, rather than work against you, and find an accountability partner whom you can meet with regularly to keep each other on track.

2. Set up a ready alternative or a displacement habit.

"A nail is driven out by another nail. Habit is overcome by habit."

—Desiderius Erasmus, Christian philosopher

A good way to break a temptation is to create an alternative attraction or activity. This is called creating a *displacement*.

How does this happen? Instead of watching a TV show in the evening after work, you could set up a regular entertaining evening activity like playing table tennis, chess, or another constructive game. If your new habit is food-related, perhaps forgo the chocolate and grab an apple or some nuts.

The point is that you want to find displacement actions that are planned rather than spontaneous. These alternate options should exclude the opportunity for temptation.

For those who eat in distress for comfort rather than hunger, which is not uncommon, listening to relaxing, preferred songs while doing things around the house can help keep them away from food. The joy from music replaces the joy from food.

3. Pay attention and choose the right time.

Most of the time, temptations come in waves. These waves can last minutes and sometimes only seconds. The good news is that, typically, temptations do not last for hours. But you must know yourself well. Learn to locate your caving point—the time when you cease to resist an urge. Once you are aware of this point, you can intentionally grab a redirecting opportunity beforehand.

So before reaching your caving point, learn to pause and find a better alternative or displacement habit. Otherwise, you may very well give in.

4. Get out of the beginning phase quickly.

Begin with easy, baby steps that you can't say no to, but do not stop there. Move past the initial stage as soon as possible. The beginning phase is usually the most unrewarding. That's why gaining proficiency at an activity is important—to get out of the rookie phase. That's when the enjoyment and benefits become apparent.

Take playing tennis as an example. Perhaps you know that initial struggle if you've tried such sports. However, once skills are acquired and mastered, sports become easier and more fun. The same principle applies to any health-related lifestyle adjustment. Try to push through during that start-up stage; the habit will become more enjoyable soon. After a month, you may even wonder why it seemed so hard!

5. Create specific goals and keep track of them.

There are countless planners to help you track nearly every-thing—from meals to exercise to daily meditation. Can't find a planner to suit your needs? You can always make one yourself instead. You will want to create a scorecard to record your daily progress. (Be sure to check out the bullet journaling system if interested.) Then, each day, you can mark that you completed the task. Share your planner with somebody else to increase accountability.

For example, runners often make a shoe-shaped grid and divide it into boxes for each day of the month, coloring each box for the days they ran. Runners can frequently track their time or mileage this way. If you get creative, you can find an enjoyable way to monitor your goals and habits. There are also phone apps that can track and inform about your daily habits.

6. Add the new habit to a good, established one.

After each cardio workout, take a cold plunge or shower. After showering daily, you can also do your ten-minute morning stretching exercises. When you brush your teeth in the morning, make a point to take your pills or supplements right afterward. That way, you won't forget to take them.

7. Set your watch five minutes faster so you arrive on time without rushing.

Developing the habit of leaving five to ten minutes earlier instead of rushing to avoid being late can have a ripple effect on other areas of our lives. Doing so can directly combat procrastination, which often stems subconsciously from a desire for an adrenaline rush. It's crucial not to rely on adrenaline as it can become addictive and create tolerance over time, much like a drug.

8. Move from a vicious circle to a positive, self-propelled one.

Have you noticed that when you exercise, you sleep better? And when you sleep better, you have more energy the next day and are more likely to exercise again? Or the opposite, when you don't move, you have less energy and do not sleep that well. That makes you less likely to exercise, so the circle goes on. Interestingly, often, both positive and vicious circles are self-propelled. Identify the negative vicious circles and replace them with positive ones. It happens with eating a lot of sweets and carbs, which pushes you into a hunger roller coaster and carbs addiction, a vicious circle. Eating low-carb, high-fat, medium-protein foods is not addictive and can replace the carbs, moving you into the positive circle where hunger disappears. Instead of snacking on crackers, cookies, or even fruit, snack on meat jerkies, prosciutto, or nuts.

9. Build the ultimate habit: Learn to get comfortable with the uncomfortable.

"Glory in our sufferings, knowing that suffering produces endurance, and endurance produces character."

—Romans 5:3-5

Champions in any field have made a habit of doing what others find boring or uncomfortable. These champions have developed strong willpower to create these new habits. Our choices should be grounded in our will (reason), not our emotions (faulty human nature). We must learn how to tolerate the uncomfortable. This is precisely the practice that successful athletes apply daily.

When you begin a new activity, try to visualize the long-term results that will come from the habit. Each of us is born with different capacities for tolerating emotional and physical hardship; however, we can improve this with experience and training.

The better we handle discomfort, the greater joy we have in life. If our focus on higher purposes becomes clouded by superficial noise, we will end up deviating, distracted, even lost, often filled with disappointment.

Minor inconveniences may prevent us from enjoying all that life has to offer. For instance, maybe you don't enjoy going to the beach because of all the sand it brings in. If this keeps you away, you'll miss out on the fantastic experiences the shore offers! In the same way, if you don't like dogs because of their shedding or their need for attention, you'll undoubtedly miss out on having a loyal four-legged companion.

Even when learning new activities such as skiing or surfing, our poor attitude toward being uncomfortable and failing may prevent us from progressing to a level where we can fully enjoy them. That's why we must learn how to be comfortable with the uncomfortable as we embrace all that life has to offer.

Consider the last time you intentionally experienced discomfort for growth, not out of obligation or need but *out of choice*. This means placing yourself in an uncomfortable situation voluntarily to reap future rewards. If more than a couple of days have passed without intentionally pushing yourself out of your comfort zone, it may be time to reassess your direction. Challenge yourself daily to do something constructive and watch as you grow. This approach can be applied to all aspects of life, including relationships.

"Pain pays the income of each precious thing."
—William Shakespeare

In summary:

Implementing good healthy habits to replace harmful ones is the most efficient way to align our lifestyle with our inherited design successfully. We can do that by applying the following concepts:

- Our body is designed to respond and adapt to persisting demands and stimulation.
- Changing the status quo and old habits is naturally resisted, but it can be done if approached in the right way.
- It requires a multidisciplinary approach that includes proper understanding and motivation, replacement habits, and resetting our values.
- Having others involved in this process greatly increases the chance of success.

In the next eight chapters, I will explore in depth the most important challenging habits you should practice on a regular basis to help you achieve true, complete health and well-being. Most of these habits were practiced by our ancestors, so they have passed the test of time and are reliable and proven to work.

Chapter 3

Intermittent Fasting

*Switching the body's fuel from sugar to ketones boosts
health and performance.*

Of the three common challenges, lack of food, cold exposure,
and strenuous physical activity, humanity has always had to deal
with, which put us in a beneficial survival state, the state of
fasting has the most profound effect on our bodies. It has a wide
range of benefits as it can be extended from a few days to a
couple of weeks.

Intermittent fasting involves taking breaks from eating for
twenty-four hours or more. Caloric intake is prohibited; only
water and unsweetened and unflavored coffee or tea are allowed
and strongly recommended. The long-term goal is to fast
twenty-four hours or more, at least one day a week. That is the
minimum required to reap some benefits. I recommend
skipping dinner and breakfast the next morning, so no food
from lunch to lunch the next day. The longer and the more
often you fast, the more significant the benefits are. Fasting for
at least an entire day causes our primary body fuel to be
switched from sugar (coming from primarily carbohydrates and
proteins) to ketones, which come from body fat.

The way our ancestors ate comprised intermittent, random
periods of involuntary fasting, as food was scarce, alternating
with periods of having one to three meals a day. Those fasting

periods would often range from one to multiple days, occasionally weeks. We should try to mimic this pattern but with shorter periods of fasting.

Fasting has many benefits, both long-term and short-term. These benefits may not manifest the first few times you fast, in the beginning, because it takes a little time to get used to it. The most important short-term benefits are increased energy and mind clarity, better sleep, improved mood, and some weight loss. Long-term benefits include those as well as more significant weight loss, reduced insulin resistance, improved digestion, reduced inflammation, slowed aging, extended lifespan, and many more. Since ancient times, sustained intermittent fasting has been practiced in most cultures and religions. Modern science studies have also shown it produces one of the most potent beneficial effects on mental and physical health.

When we prolong our fasting periods, we place a demand on our bodies to mobilize inner resources. These include genetic adaptation and performance enhancement mechanisms because we switch to hunting or survival mode, with significant added benefits described earlier in the book. A study by the Queen Mary University of London found that a seven-day fast can trigger a multi-organ response, demonstrating health benefits that extend way beyond simple weight loss.

Basic intermittent fasting.

Fasting is like muscle-building: the more you train, the stronger it becomes. This is not a process to rush. You must begin with baby steps. If you continue, then you will eventually reap great results. To begin, skip one meal for one or two days a week. Avoid eating anything between meals during this time. Also, remember to drink plenty of water while fasting. This is extremely important.

I highly recommend skipping dinner rather than breakfast or lunch. You don't have enough time after dinner to burn the calories you ingest before bed. So, going to bed with those excess calories can lead to weight gain since the body must transform the surge of calories into fat storage. Plus, when skipping the last meal, you will be asleep when you are hungriest.

If you can skip dinner once or twice weekly for a few weeks, you will become more comfortable with this practice. Then you can skip the second meal—breakfast. You will only drink water (which contains zero calories) from lunch the first day to lunch the next day.

The water should have minerals, as regular commercial bottled water has low mineral content. We should add naturally sourced minerals to all the water we drink. This type of fasting is the bare minimum and should continue throughout the year for most of your life. After all, you can't say you don't have time to skip dinner, right?

At first, if you're stressed or tired, then I do not recommend fasting. Choose a regular, full workday to begin on instead. This will allow time to pass faster, and you won't have much opportunity to think about food.

After fasting for a couple of months—at least twenty-four-hour intervals once or twice a week—the metabolic mechanisms of the switch from sugar to ketones will become fully functional. This fulfills our inherited genetic design. Our ancestors endured thousands of years of fasting since food was scarce and difficult to find, so we are perfectly adapted to this shift in fuel. We perform far better when fasting because the survival mechanisms kick into gear, enabling us to hunt or find food.

Unfortunately, we are still cavemen, genetically speaking. We still have a strong hunger drive. Consider the fact that it is usually far easier to gain weight than it is to lose weight. Why? Because until recently (less than two hundred years ago), people had lived in survival mode for thousands of years. When they found food, they ate as much as possible to gain fat that could provide the calories to survive until food was found again.

Advanced intermittent fasting.

After a while, many people find twenty-four-hour fasting intervals to be very rewarding, so they fast twenty-four hours four or five days during the week. These people will only eat between noon and two in the afternoon and only have dinner and breakfast on the weekends.

Once you are comfortable fasting for twenty-four hours, you can skip a third meal. Here's an example: At this point, you may decide only to eat lunch on Monday. Then you will eat again at dinner on Tuesday evening. Thirty hours will pass without food consumption. I challenge you to practice this thirty-hour fast once a week for a few weeks or alternate it with twenty-four-hour fasts.

At this point, the brain fully accepts ketones as an energy source and no longer craves sugar as caloric intake. There is a large reserve of ketones from body fat. The metabolic mechanism of switching from sugars to ketones becomes fully functional.

A long-term goal is to fast at least one or two days a week (continuously or intermittently) for most of your life. Some people may advance to three consecutive days a week quarterly and even seven consecutive days once a year. However, even a few months of fasting, one or two days a week, can positively affect your energy, mood, mental clarity, and inflammatory symptoms. These positive results will hopefully motivate you to carry on with this practice.

Frequent fasting can make the transition between the two fuels (carbs/sugars and ketones) smoother, easier, and faster. This, in return, will help you feel less hungry when your blood sugar is dropping. Your body would be happy to use your own fat much sooner, even before it uses the stored sugar.

As previously mentioned, fasting can also shrink the stomach, causing you to feel satisfied and full quicker than usual. This, of course, reduces the amount of food you eat. A small stomach is a critical factor in weight loss, reducing stomach acid, and improving flora and digestion.

When animals fast, they tend to become more agile, faster, and sharper because they have no choice but to find food or hunt. This is when their survival mechanisms kick into gear. We, too, tend to perform the best when our bodies rely on ketones as fuel instead of sugar. The opposite is also true: We usually perform the worst *after* meals, especially after eating a lot of carbs.

Potential issues and common failures.

Uncomfortable symptoms.

During the first few fasting experiences, you may face a variety of uncomfortable symptoms aside from the expected hunger pains. These symptoms may range from mood changes and agitation to headaches and stomach pains. These side effects are both typical and expected. The reason is the body's and brain's reluctance to switch fuel from external sources to sugar reserves and then to fat. So, what should you do when these symptoms arise?

First, take baby steps and be consistent. Perhaps you can omit just one meal at first—dinner. Do this every week, at least twice a week, without skipping to prevent the body from having to readjust, and you will learn quicker.

To make it easier, eat a low-carb meal before the fasting period begins, like eggs with avocado, cheese, and bacon. A high-carb meal is followed by a rise in blood sugar level, followed by a stronger insulin response, which eventually reduces the blood sugar significantly after that. This sudden drop in blood sugar sends powerful triggers of hunger and related symptoms, so we crave carbs and sugar and end up on a reactive-eating roller coaster. That eventually leads to insulin resistance. That means increasing insulin levels are required to do the same job, to reduce the elevated sugar. Unfortunately, insulin makes you gain weight.

Overeating after fasting.

To prevent overeating after fasting, try to apply the conscious eating technique of eating slowly and chewing well as is described in detail in Chapter 6. Even after you fast for sixteen hours, your stomach will shrink and incite a quicker feeling of fullness. Problems can arise due to a five-to-ten-minute delay between becoming full and our brains recognizing this signal. This can cause us to feel still hungry, even when the stomach is physically full—and this, in return, can cause us to overeat.

Remember that embracing discomfort is a necessary part of the process. We must endure these challenges for much more rewarding and delayed gratification.

Historical background.

Before the Industrial Revolution, food shortages forced most people to fast involuntarily. Even today, in most developing nations, most people lack enough food to consume daily. Our typical way of eating—with short breaks that last only four to six hours—is unnatural, new only to Western civilization and in modern times.

Fasting is mentioned in many written sources, regardless of religion, geographical location, or race. These sources suggest that this method has proven its effectiveness throughout the centuries. This practice was used by many physicians, philosophers, and priests in ancient Egypt, India, and Greece for curative and preventive purposes or as a means of strengthening the spirit.

In the Bible, numerous verses advise fasting solely for spiritual reasons:

"I humbled my soul with fasting" (Psalm 35:13, NAS).

"Jesus, full of the Holy Spirit, returned from the Jordan and was led by the spirit in the desert, where the devil tempted him for forty days. He ate nothing during those days, and at the end of them, he was hungry" (Luke 4:1-2, NIV).

"But when you fast, put oil on your head and wash your face, so that it will not be obvious to men that you are fasting, but only to your Father, who is unseen; and your Father, who sees what is done in secret, will reward you" (Matthew 6:17-18 NIV).

Pythagoras (580–500 BC)—Greek philosopher, mathematician, and founder of the famous school of philosophy—regularly fasted for forty days, believing it increased mental perception and creativity. He required each of his disciples and followers to adhere to a strict fast of forty days on water alone.

Plato (427–347, BCE), a disciple of Socrates, was a Greek philosopher who divided medicine into "true," which brings health, and "false," which brings only the "phantom of health." The first one included treatment of fasting and dieting, air, and sunshine.

Hippocrates (460–357 BC) was a physician known as the founder of the medical commandment that states, "Do no harm." He was also an ardent supporter of moderation and treatment through fasting. He wrote:

"The addition of food should be much rarer since it is often useful to completely take it away while the patient can withstand it until the force of the disease reaches its maturity. The man carries within him a doctor; you just have to help him do his work. If the body is not cleared, then the more you feed it, the more it will be harmed. When a patient is fed too richly, the disease is fed as well. Remember—any excess is against nature."

Hippocrates, Galen, and Paracelsus, the three fathers of Western medicine, fasted and prescribed the same treatments to their patients. Paracelsus concluded nearly five hundred years ago: "Fasting is the greatest remedy—the physician within!"

Since we are shaped after the way our ancestors lived, we are genetically designed to fast. As mentioned earlier, we are also designed to gain weight and possess a strong hunger drive that serves as a primary survival mechanism. As humankind advanced, we could obtain food more easily—but for most of us, one full meal per day was a luxury. This was typical until the Industrial Revolution when food became abundant. We are naturally designed to eat once a day or less for these reasons.

Science and further reasoning.

A substantial amount of research supports the health benefits of fasting.

Some recent studies have found that increasing the time between meals improves the overall health of male mice and increases their lifespan compared to mice who eat more frequently. Perhaps even more surprisingly, these health benefits were seen regardless of what the mice ate or how many calories they consumed.

It's also been proven that fasting can improve disease biomarkers, reduce oxidative stress, and preserve learning and memory function. Experts in the field have developed several theories to explain why fasting provides physiological benefits. For example, there is a hypothesis that cells experience mild stress during fasting. It also states that they respond adaptively to stress by enhancing their ability to cope with stress and possibly resist disease.

Though the word *stress* is often used negatively, it can produce benefits. Consider, for example, vigorous exercise. This may momentarily stress your muscles and the cardiovascular system, but over time, your muscles will grow stronger as the body recovers and continues to exercise.

"There is considerable similarity between how cells respond to the stress of exercise and how cells respond to intermittent fasting," explains Mark Mattson, a science professor specializing in fasting. Mattson has also researched the protective benefits of fasting on neurons, including protection of memory, and learning functionality and slowing disease processes in the brain.

Nature's wisdom uses fasting as a defense mechanism against infection. Losing one's appetite is an instinctual way for both animals and men to defend against the bacteria that require the energy and nutrients from our food.

Fasting causes our bodies to switch the fuel source from external (glucose from food) to internal (ketones). When we fast, our low sugar levels cause our bodies to switch to ketones as an energy source, which most bacteria and yeast cannot use. After twelve to twenty-four hours of zero caloric intake, the sugar stored in the liver and muscles becomes exhausted (this depends on the individual consumption rate). First, the muscles and then the brain must accept ketones as fuel instead of sugar. Ketones result from the breakdown of fat, either our own or ingested. This is a common situation that both animals and humans alike have experienced over thousands of years. Therefore, we became genetically programmed to do this.

After fasting for more than twenty-four hours, we enter a ketogenic state known as *ketosis*. You may have heard of the "ketogenic diet" before, as it is increasingly gaining popularity and success. This diet keeps the individual in a ketosis state because the meals contain almost zero carbs, high amounts of healthy fat, and moderate amounts of proteins.

It's important to note that fasting is different from starvation. When someone is starving, they break down their own proteins from muscle to produce glucose. The conversion of the body's structural proteins into glucose as the primary energy source occurs when no more fat is available to convert into ketones.

Most of us have over twenty percent body fat. The average in the U.S. is around twenty-eight percent among men and forty percent among women. That means we would have enough fuel to endure more than a week of complete fasting without entering starvation.

At first, changing fuel types is a challenge, especially for the brain. But if you follow an intermittent and progressive process of changing fuels weekly, your body will soon adapt. The body will ease into the change and get used to it within a few months. Then, the initial discomfort that most people experience will significantly diminish. As switching from sugar to ketones becomes more natural, especially when you fast more often, your brain will begin to adapt easily and quickly.

Another benefit of fasting is the psychological aspect. In addition to entering a clearer state of mind and mental well-being, fasting brings your attention to possible poor eating habits, such as eating out of boredom or stress. Fasting strengthens your willpower and improves your discipline, which everyone could benefit from.

As you can imagine, this discipline, although not always "easy" to adapt, can radically transform your life.

In summary:

Intermittent fasting involves abstaining from any food or caloric intake for at least twenty-four hours, at least one day a week. During the fasting period, you may drink water, unflavored tea, or coffee. Longer fasting periods of multiple days are even more beneficial.

It is recommended to add minerals to the water during fasting to avoid any deficiencies.

Intermittent fasting has multiple benefits, including weight loss, reduced insulin resistance, improved digestion, body detoxing, improved mental capabilities, and life extension.

Chapter 4

Cold Water, Sauna, and Contrast Temperatures Practices

Push your body into survival mode with multiple immediate and long-term health benefits.

Exposing yourself to more extreme temperatures is another efficient and readily available method to challenge and stimulate your body and mobilize your inner resources for healing and regenerating. Both cold water plunges and hot saunas have stood the test of time. They have been practiced as health treatments for thousands of years in multiple cultures, particularly in Scandinavian countries, Russia, Japan, and Korea.

I recently had a healthy middle-aged woman as a patient who had lost her father a couple of months ago. She could not function, sleep, or even eat right. She was very attached to her father, and his death was unexpected and sudden. She was crying most of the day. Despite support from family and mourning therapy, two months later, she was worse.

She came to me for help, and although she didn't like drugs, she was ready to start something. I suggested she do a daily cold plunge in an unheated pool, which would be in the 50s in winter in Florida. I explained to her the benefits and mentioned two British studies that showed significant improvement in depressed patients practicing the cold plunges. I prescribed a few low-dose clonazepam pills, an anti-anxiety medication, for situations when she had to function.

I gave her detailed instructions on how to start the cold therapy gradually. A month later, she came back significantly improved. She had barely touched the clonazepam pills. At the time of the second visit, she had already been swimming for fifteen minutes daily in the 54-degree pool.

Cold water plunges, also known as *cold therapy*, can provide significant health benefits. Cold showers are an acceptable alternative, although they are less powerful and less efficient. Here are some of the most notable benefits of cold therapy:

Increased circulation: When exposed to cold water, blood vessels constrict and expand as the body heats up. This process creates a flash of blood effect, increasing blood flow and circulation, reducing muscle soreness, and aiding injury recovery.

Increased vitality and alertness: A cold-water soak stimulates the body to increase feelings of energy and alertness. Practicing this method habitually can also help improve mood and reduce symptoms of depression and anxiety.

Reduced inflammation: Cold water immersion can help reduce inflammation in the body, especially in joints and muscles, helping to reduce swelling and pain. The exact mechanism still needs to be fully understood.

Improved immune function: Cold water immersion can also help improve immune function by increasing the production of white blood cells responsible for fighting off infections and illnesses. There are numerous people who, upon taking one cold water plunge, will go months without developing a common cold. The incidence of common colds is also significantly reduced in cold-water swimmers.

Improved post-workout recovery: Cold water immersion can help reduce muscle soreness and aid post-workout recovery. It also helps reduce the risk of injury by increasing flexibility and range of motion. (This is due to its after-effect of reducing inflammation and increasing blood flow.)

Improved skin and hair health: Cold water helps to tighten and firm the skin, reducing the appearance of pores and fine lines. It can also improve hair health by increasing blood flow to the scalp.

However, it is essential to note that cold water immersion can be dangerous for some people, especially those with underlying health conditions such as asthma. Be sure to consult with a healthcare professional before attempting it. It is also recommended to start with short sessions first and gradually increase the duration. You can transform your bathtub into a cold plunge system by purchasing a water chiller for well below $1,000, or you can put ice and water in it.

Sauna benefits.

The effects of heat increase our circulation and oxygen supply to peripheral tissues by dilating blood vessels. When we sweat, toxins such as harmful metabolites and heavy metals are expelled through the skin.

Heat has a powerful effect on relaxing muscles, ligaments, and joints. It also improves stiffness and pain in areas of chronic inflammation, such as injuries and arthritis.

Taking saunas is also a great way to relax and disconnect. As you deal with the physiological changes in your body caused by rising temperatures, you have no choice but to remain focused on the moment. This is an excellent opportunity to meditate and observe how your body reacts to rising temperatures.

There are many different types of saunas, each with specific benefits beyond the general benefits listed above. In addition to detoxification, the moisture provided in a steam sauna helps to clear sinuses and improve respiratory health. Adding herbs and essential oils to a wet sauna can enhance the many benefits of aromatherapy.

Compared to other health measures, such as dietary changes and exercise, the health benefits of extreme temperature exposures are striking and can be felt immediately. They produce a strong and positive mental response that amplifies their benefits.

Sauna—your first few sessions.

You will need your physician's approval before beginning cold-water plunges or sauna practices. Saunas are not good for certain health conditions, such as high fever and diarrhea with dehydration. Also, I don't recommend the sauna contrast method for people who are just starting out. This contrast method is also not recommended for individuals with asthma, as rapid contrast can trigger an asthma attack.

Not everyone can tolerate saunas at first. Beginners may experience dizziness, lightheadedness, fatigue, feeling excessively hot, or increased heart rate. If you experience these or any other unpleasant symptoms, get out of the sauna and don't return until the next day.

Key points to remember:
- To help prevent an unpleasant experience, ensure proper hydration for a few days before the sauna. If you wait until you are thirsty, you are already dehydrated. Consuming at least the average amount of water, which is sixty-four ounces per day, is advised. However, the needed amount will vary significantly based on climate, temperature, location, humidity, activity level, and so on. You must also ensure you have enough electrolytes, as you will lose a lot while sweating. You should add minerals to your water and eat saltier foods. Make sure

to get plenty of rest. I also advise eating a healthy meal (low in carbs and high in healthy fats) a few hours before your first sauna session.

- Going to the sauna too late in the evening may be too energizing and can disturb your sleep. You may want to experiment to see if this applies to you.

- Be sure to weigh yourself first. Hopefully, you will weigh the same after your sauna session is complete. If you don't, then you are dehydrated. To regain your pre-sauna weight, you will need to drink plenty of water with minerals.

- Wear cotton shirts (either short- or long-sleeved) and pants (short or long). This helps absorb some of the sweat and prevents the toxic chemicals from being reabsorbed back through your skin. If you are sensitive to heat, wear a sauna hat to protect your head from the heat.

- Start with a low temperature—say about 130 F. Wet saunas are usually more difficult to tolerate than dry saunas.

- Drink water in the sauna before you get thirsty.

- Watch for signs that you are feeling "off." Get out immediately if this occurs.

- Be aware that you may feel lightheaded or dizzy when standing up. When you stand, do so slowly and against the wall. Please do not enter the sauna in the dark, as it may cause dizziness and lightheadedness.

- Concentrate on your breathing. Breathe slowly and use your abdominal muscles.

- You can use the sauna for up to fifteen minutes the first few times. Then, you can gradually increase the duration and temperature.

Contrast hot to cold.

Temperature contrasts, accomplished by going straight from a sauna into the cold, shock the body. This is a powerful and effective technique that provides many combined benefits. It only feels aggressive at first. But if it is practiced consistently—at least two to three times a week—after the first three to four sessions, the severity of discomfort diminishes quickly.

Pushing your body outside your comfort zone through extreme temperature exposures, especially when repeated over time, sends powerful messages to your genetic survival mechanisms. The body doesn't know that you are doing this voluntarily. It puts you in a "survival mode" (as explained in previous chapters), and this mode improves health and general performance. The specific mechanisms of how this happens are not well understood, nor is it required to take advantage of the practices.

Contrast, cold water plunges or cold shower practice.

Start using the contrast method only after you have taken a few sauna sessions; that way, you will be more accustomed to the high temperatures.

The most effective treatment is to plunge fully into a frigid bath. But if this is not available, a frigid shower is the next best thing. A bucket of cold water is also effective. If you cannot tolerate exposing your body to the cold, put your head underneath a cold shower instead. While doing this, you can imagine basking in the sun on a beach or a tropical island.

You can apply the contrast method more than once during longer sauna sessions. Only do as many contrast sessions as you feel you can handle.

A warning: Do not apply the contrast method if you feel weak or tired. Only do this when you feel in good condition.

Hot and cold showers.

When you don't go to the sauna or if you don't have access to one, I recommend practicing a contrast temperature shower as an alternative.

Start with moderate temperatures and gradually increase to extreme temperatures. First, take a warm shower, then change the temperature to hot for a few minutes. Try to expose all parts of the body to it. Then, change the temperature to cold and stand underneath the cold water for about twenty seconds. This may shock your system initially but try to remain beneath the cold water for twenty seconds. If this is too much, you can ease your body into it instead by initially turning the water to cold gradually. Limit the cold sessions to less than one minute. Your goal, however, should be to contrast the water temperature and quickly change it from hot to cold. This method provides the most benefits. You may feel like screaming or jumping around at the beginning. That's normal, but the unpleasant sensation should dissipate soon as your body adjusts to the temperature change.

Then, you can turn the water back to warm and stay underneath the warm water for an additional few minutes. Repeat for a couple of cycles, gradually increasing the time you spend beneath the cold water. Try to spend at least twice as long in hot water as in cold water.

End your shower with a final blast of cold water to invigorate your body.

Other recommendations.

After a sauna, you should shower with soap and shampoo your hair. If possible, brush your teeth and tongue. You want to remove all the toxins accumulated on the surface of your body from sweating. Then, weigh yourself to make sure you're not dehydrated. If you weigh less than before entering the sauna, drink water with electrolytes until you regain the pre-sauna weight.

Afterward, eat a light meal and take it easy. Avoid intense physical activity and relax or sleep.

Try to go to the sauna at least once a week, ideally with the contrast method applied.

You can also contrast every time you shower.

While exposed to cold, do not stay completely still. Move your arms and legs if you can. The ideal cold plunge is to swim slowly in freezing water.

The use of cold water, sauna, and contrast temperatures is another excellent, healthy challenge and willpower exercise. It will test and improve your capacity to deal with discomfort. Remarkably, the rewards are often felt immediately and are more evident than the delayed ones. But the immediate benefits don't typically last for more than a few hours. If you develop this into a regular habit, you will reap significant long-term health benefits.

In summary:

Cold therapy plunges involve immersing yourself in cold water or taking a cold shower for a few minutes regularly, at least three to four times per week. It is recommended to gradually introduce yourself to cold therapy by starting with 70 or 60°F water and gradually reducing the temperature to ideally 40 or even 30s°F.

Cold plunges are designed to shock and make you uncom-fortable. This is a challenge that puts your body in survival mode with multiple immediate and long-term benefits. It will invigorate and energize you immediately, and in the long term, can improve your mood, reduce depression and anxiety, and improve your sleep. In addition, cold therapy can also reduce inflammation, improve immunity and resistance to colds, and help you lose weight.

A hot sauna involves spending a minimum of fifteen minutes in high temperatures between 130 and 190°F. It is also recommended to start gradually with respect to time and temperature. It has multiple benefits, including detoxing through sweating, physical and mental relaxation, and improving stiffness and pain in areas of chronic inflammation, such as injuries and arthritis.

Chapter 5

Exercising, Stretching, and Playing

How to discover and use our nearly unlimited healing capacities through movement for a high-quality and rewarding life.

The response to the physical demands that we accomplish by stimulating our body through different exercises goes far beyond burning calories, losing weight, and mechanically stimulating our vascular system and different parts of our body. There are profound positive reactions in our minds, emotions, and genes.

That explains why exercise is a powerful way to reduce the incidence of vascular disease, including heart attack and stroke, cancer, and Alzheimer's disease simultaneously.

This chapter focuses on activities that push you out of your comfort zone and create a significant demand that awakens your inner resources to respond and adapt to become healthier, physically, and mentally. Whether doing cardio exercise, stretching, or weightlifting, you will measure your heart rate to achieve the above purpose, reflecting the degree of effort necessary to achieve this goal.

When you engage in intense exercises, your body naturally detoxes and protects you from excessive inflammation. This occurs when you sweat and when the activities increase blood flow through your body's organs. This process flushes out toxins and waste that your metabolism has produced. Because more intense exercise involves some degree of muscle and soft tissue destruction and inflammation, this contributes to regeneration and helps to strengthen those tissues.

Exercise doesn't need to be dreadful. Why not make it fun? It's a powerful tool that can help you disconnect and reset from the stresses of your daily life.

By exercising, you are focused on acknowledging your weaknesses rather than ignoring them. The result is that you grow stronger and healthier.

These physical challenges allow your potential and inner strength to become unleashed. They strengthen your will, your discipline, and your resilience.

Your intimate life, sexual well-being, and performance can be dramatically improved by starting a habitual sustained exercise program. Vigorous exercise improves sexual hormone levels, reduces stress, and increases libido and the sense of well-being. It disconnects you from stress and makes you more joyful.

There is likely a direct connection between the quality of living and duration of your life. One related factor is the heart rate. What if we are born with a limited, maximum number of heartbeats for a lifetime, which would be genetically inherited? How we preserve or waste our heartbeats would depend on the quality of our lives. Regular activities such as exercise, meditation, and good quality sleep reduce the number of daily heartbeats, and they are extending our lifespan, also demonstrated scientifically. In contrast, persistent stress, suffering, and poor conditioning increase our average daily number of heartbeats, and they are shortening our lives. Most athletes have low resting heart rates, indicating their good health. Things that reduce the number of daily heartbeats are going to prolong our lives and, not coincidentally, are also improving life quality.

The Practice.

Ask your physician if you are cleared to do cardio exercises. Start with at least two hours a week of cardio, split into two or three sessions. You can achieve cardio-level exercise by doing active stretching or weightlifting; you need to reach the heart rate goal described below. The best way is to measure your heart rate with a sports watch or other devices.

If your resting heart rate per minute falls between 60 BPM (beats per minute) and 80 BPM, which it is in most of us, then see the formula below that explains the heart rate goal:

Maximum heart rate should be 220 BPM minus your age.

To illustrate this, let's say you are fifty years old. Subtract fifty from 220, and you will find that your maximum heart rate should be 170 BPM. You should alternate and change the pace, as with one-minute intense followed by two-minute moderate effort.

During your intense minutes of exercise, your heart rate should be between seventy and ninety percent of the max of 170 BPM. That would fall somewhere in the 120s to140s range. Your heart rate should be between 100 and 120 BPM for moderate intervals.

Age = 50

Max heart rate = 220 - 50 = 170 BPM

The heart rate during intense intervals of exercise should be between 120 and 140 BPM (approximately 80%).

The heart rate for moderate intervals should be between 100 and 120 BPM.

The more you exercise and increase your heart rate, the lower your heart rate will be while resting, resulting in a lower total number of heartbeats daily.

You should incorporate interval-intensity training into your workouts. You alternate between more intense training and less intense *intervals* in these workouts. (I will explain the benefits of this later in this chapter.) Here's an example of this type of exercise: You would run faster for one minute and jog slower for two minutes. Any exercise machine cardio program will have this interval option on its menu. Your heart rate goal for the faster running minute should be seventy to ninety percent of your maximum heart rate. Your goal for the slower jogging two minutes should be sixty to seventy percent of your maximum heart rate.

These intervals occur naturally and spontaneously in a sport such as tennis, basketball, or volleyball.

Start exercising with somebody else. You need to set yourself accountable, at least until it becomes a habit.

The best way to start a new exercise or stretching habit is to involve somebody else. You need to have some form of accountability to prevent you from skipping or cheating without consequences. One way to do this is by paying for a class. Investing in an exercise class or a personal trainer may be one of the wisest investments. We should also choose activities that we like, as well as exercises that fit our age and our body condition. Individuals who are markedly overweight should avoid, or at least limit, impactful weight-bearing exercises.

We need to trade remote, unavoidable pain for immediate voluntary discomfort.

There's no denying that if you attempt a cardio exercise that involves increasing heart rates to your BPM goals, you will experience some degree of discomfort. This may especially be true at the beginning of the exercise. During these moments, let's be determined not to give up. You can trust that there will be many significant rewards to follow. Most of these rewards, however, are rather *remote* instead of immediate. But each of us needs to learn how to become a *good trader.*

You can learn to trade a significantly higher, delayed, and unavoidable suffering—like the price of developing obesity, diabetes, or cardiovascular disease—for immediate and less painful discomfort. The type of discomfort that only comes when you push yourself out of your comfort zone to reach your heart rate goal. Choose your challenge and pain and stay in control, or they will choose you.

Make it fun play.

Even if physical activity isn't a game, why not have fun? *Playing* gives you the freedom to enjoy life. If you approach exercise with this mindset, you will likely be more motivated to continue the habit long-term. There's nothing wrong with playing. All animals and humans have found ways to have fun from the very beginning of time.

Playing can teach necessary life lessons—such as how to handle both winning and losing. You also learn how to deal with your pride and ego. It allows you to connect with people, even those different from you, work with them as a team, and ultimately form connections. Playing sports unites people as they work toward a common goal and learn to deal with conflict and negative emotions.

I also emphasize the benefits of playing table tennis (commonly known as Ping-Pong). One study published in the *Encyclopedia Journal* has shown that Ping-Pong is one of the most potent ways to prevent dementia and Alzheimer's. The demand to react quickly, focus, and concentrate stimulates the brain through genetic protective mechanisms, even if the heart rate goal is not always achieved. When these mechanisms are stimulated, performance increases. This is another example of a high-demand activity that results in a positive response from our body. By mimicking activities and survival movements, Ping-Pong offers several health benefits. The best part is that this is an easy activity that offers minimal risk of injuries.

Make sure you stretch well and warm up before exercising.

One way to avoid an injury is to stretch frequently. It is especially crucial to prioritize stretching as the body ages since it grows stiffer. As mentioned earlier, stiffness can be dangerous during intense exercise. The stiffer your body becomes, the greater the chances of an injury.

You must actively stretch for a minimum of five minutes, ideally ten or more, before engaging in physical activities to prevent injuries and increase performance. Active stretching means active movement with a range of motion of different body parts. It is recommended over passive stretching at the beginning of the exercise. You also should do passive stretching at the end of a workout to reduce muscle soreness and improve recovery.

Chi-gong is a complete way to exercise and achieve well-being. One of the best ways to stretch, unrelated to warm up, especially for people over fifty, is to do chi-gong and tai chi. The Chinese have practiced these movements for thousands of years; therefore, they have stood the test of time well enough to be considered safe and reliable.

Chi-gong is a gentler approach to active stretching that also results in more significant benefits. These movements stimulate internal organs, improve balance, and sharpen concentration. More intense variations of chi-gong and tai chi can be considered a full cardio workout.

Yoga is another ancient and time-proof method of static stretching that improves overall well-being. This is also widely practiced in the West, but caution must be applied when engaging in yoga to prevent injury. It's especially vital to be careful if you are stiff.

Even if you do not practice the same spirituality as these Eastern cultures, you can still benefit from their approaches to health. You can maintain your own spiritual beliefs while focusing on these commonalities.

The positive genetic response to the demand to exercise.

For thousands of years, the law of nature was this: If we didn't move, we died—just like in the animal world. Yet our modern technology now affords us to be sedentary. That is very destructive for both our physical and our mental health. We must learn to live in alignment with our design. We were designed to move, lift, carry, run, fight, and hunt, just as our ancestors did for thousands of years. This is *survival 101*. Frequent strenuous activities, such as aerobic exercises, send messages to the body's genetic adaptation mechanisms to adapt to the demands. These are similar to the demands that require us to survive.

Our bodies and genes don't know that we are not in a struggle for survival. The body can't recognize that you are doing these exercises for different survival purposes. Your body's response to these activities is genetic—for instance, the way your muscles respond to weightlifting. They grow and become stronger. These genetic responses to performance demands aren't unique to muscle building. They improve blood circulation, immunity, resilience, healing capacity, focus, and even your thinking. If you persist in these actions, your body will transform into a survivalist with enhanced performance and health. These repetitive and demanding signals to your DNA complex not only activate the "good genes" but also turn off the bad genes inherited from parents and grandparents.

So, we can see how *change will not arrive if we remain in our comfort zones*. Embracing challenges makes us stronger.

The direct physical effect of exercise on our heart and vascular system.

With all that being said, not all movements are created equal. When it comes to living longer, our two main enemies are cardiovascular disease and cancer.

How can we prevent cardiovascular disease? Exercise is the number one method. If we hope to reduce plaque formation, we must keep the arteries flexible, smooth, and healthy. We need to stimulate the blood vessels mechanically. The best way to do this is to distend and stretch the blood vessels.

There are two main methods for doing this. The most important way is to increase the size of the arteries by increasing the blood flow. We must stretch them from the inside out by increasing the diameter. How do we do this? By increasing blood flow through increasing cardiac output. During aerobic exercises, the heart rate increases significantly and pumps more blood volume per minute (cardiac output) than it does while resting. This causes the arteries to dilate, sometimes more than twice the resting diameter, to accommodate the blood flow. Regular practice of this ensures healthy blood vessels.

This can help even if a person has developed arterial blockages. The consistent, sustained demand for increased blood flow will, over time, allow the body's intelligence adaptive mechanisms to compensate for the occlusion and dilate existing smaller collateral vessels (or even create new collaterals). Then, if a narrow artery becomes completely blocked—by a blood clot, for instance—it would not lead to a heart attack or a stroke.

If you can stretch the blood vessels from the outside through methods such as yoga, chi-gong, and other stretching exercises, then you will also stimulate the blood vessels, preventing them from becoming stiff and frail.

Another benefit of stretching is that it increases the flexibility of your muscles and tendons, which can help to prevent injuries. An injury would prevent you from engaging in cardiovascular activities and likely cause you to become sedentary.

There is a strong correlation between the intensity of exercise and the number of medications one requires to take.

From my internal medicine practice, which I have practiced for over twenty-five years, I have found a close correlation between a patient's exercise level and the number of medications they take. Even among the sixty- to seventy-year-old age groups, there is a close to one hundred percent correlation between being heavily physically active and not needing to take prescription drugs. If exercise intensity decreases from heavy to moderate, most people—particularly those over fifty—would likely require at least one or two prescription drugs. If exercise is absent or only occasional in the individual's lifestyle, diabetic or cardiac pills are typically added to their daily medications.

Pick an exercise type that matches your body design.

As we exercise, we should continue to vary the intensity and the types of exercises we engage in. As I've explained, this type of movement aligns with our body's design.

Remember that the human body has already been pre-designed and shaped by the lifestyles of our ancestors. With this in mind, we must realize the harm of prolonged running on concrete. This is true even if we wear soft, thick shoe insoles.

I've met many patients in my practice who have suffered from these injuries. Our ancestors did not run at the same pace on a flat, hard surface. Instead, their running style mimicked trail running in the woods, with multiple obstacles and inclines. This type of running varies in pace as well. Sadly, most people today do not engage in this style of running. Most modern-day runners will run on the street at the same pace and speed for a long time. This can be damaging as repetitive impact becomes cumulative.

This is why I recommend changing your running pace. Doing this will protect your joints. You should also avoid hitting your heels when running and run like you are barefoot or as near barefoot as possible—which is precisely how we ran for thousands of years. This type of action forces you to take smaller steps and land on your front foot with your knees bent. This form is far more protective for the joints. Using a cardio program found in most exercise machines may also be a good idea. These programs offer the same pace and angle of impact and intensity variation.

It's ideal to alternate running exercises with other low-impact exercises, such as swimming, biking, an elliptical machine, a stepper machine, or bouncing on a trampoline. Then, you can continue to run for many years to come.

According to the pre-design theory, physical inactivity affects men more than women. This is because men have historically been more active than women. As such, the changes that result from a sedentary lifestyle tend to be more dramatic for men, leading to more severe adverse effects on the body. This also helps explain the higher incidence of heart attacks and vascular disease in men than women.

In summary:

For exercise to be fully beneficial, it needs to be challenging enough to push us into survival mode. We should aim for variable intensity intervals, totaling at least two hours each week. This involves increasing our heart rate, which should be measured and targeted based on our age, as it reflects the degree of effort.

We should also stretch regularly to prevent injuries and reap additional benefits. The benefits of exercise and stretching go beyond weight loss and improving mood and cardiovascular health to include reducing the risk of cancer and Alzheimer's disease.

Chapter 6

Conscious Eating

*Mindful eating to achieve digestive health and
lose weight.*

Conscious eating is *the way* in which one should eat. This type
of eating is not dependent on, or limited to, a particular diet. It
involves chewing food slowly and well without doing any other
activity.

A popular old saying from Chinese wisdom explains conscious eating this way: "*Drink your food and eat your drink.*"
Drinking food involves chewing the food until it becomes as soft
as baby food before swallowing. *Eating your drink* involves
sipping a liquid drink slowly, one sip at a time, and "chewing"
it much like you would chew solid food so that the liquid
mixes with your saliva and reaches your body temperature
before swallowing.

Mindful eating has many health benefits, quickly felt by
those who practice it regularly.

Chewing well and drinking slowly both significantly improve digestion. This also reduces the amount of food you eat
before feeling full and satisfied, often resulting in a smaller
stomach size and weight loss.

In addition, the practice reduces esophageal reflux and
stomach acid, increases nutrient absorption, and reduces gut
inflammation and an unhealthy overgrowth of gut bacteria.

People who practice mindful eating may also enjoy improved sleep and energy quality (more details on this at the end of this chapter).

In addition, this practice can reduce excessive gas, diarrhea, and constipation.

This practice doesn't only provide benefits for the body—it benefits the psyche as well. Our busy, fast-paced, and multitasking society has conditioned us to develop an addiction to productivity. We constantly feel as though we must be doing something. So, when we eat, it is difficult to stop everything and simply enjoy the meal. Mindful eating invites us to disconnect, slow down, and relax. It can be considered a mind exercise that can help improve attention deficit disorder and anxiety.

Basic conscious eating practice.

When you eat, sit down, and resist the temptation to do any other activity. View this time as a moment of relaxation. This means no talking, TV, electronic devices, or reading to distract from your meal. Disconnecting from daily stresses or excitement is essential, as this will reduce your sympathetic nervous system activity. (Our sympathetic nervous system is responsible for governing the fight-or-flight responses.)

During the first few weeks of adapting this practice, count how many times you chew each bite. This will prevent your mind from wandering onto something else. Chew each bite at least thirty-six times for hard-to-digest foods such as meats and raw vegetables (according to the traditional Chinese method). Chew each bite about twenty-four times when eating soft, easily digestible foods like fish, steamed vegetables, yogurt, or eggs.

At first, this practice may seem tedious. But after a few days of mindful eating, you will discover a renewed appreciation for the rest and relaxation that comes with eating. This can lead to developing an eating-meditation habit in the *advanced conscious eating practice.*

Advanced conscious eating practice.

By disconnecting from the daily "noise" and life concerns while eating, you will enter a peaceful, relaxed state similar to the calm state achieved by mindful meditation. To do this, bring your focus to the moment at hand. Focus only on the food in front of you and on your body. What is your sitting position? How full do you feel? Do you have any pressure or tightness in your body? Stay alert to each feeling of hunger. When it arises, try to follow it mentally and then notice when it subsides. You can also notice the temperature and texture of the food, the flavor of various ingredients, and how these elements change while chewing. See the Meditation chapter for more information on practicing and improving this.

Potential issues and common failures.

As long as you do not have a limitation that prevents you from chewing, then there should not be any issues that arise with this practice. All habits developed in the learning stage have similar possible causes for failure. Burnout, lack of perseverance, and lack of will are the main reasons people may not progress or see results.

Historical background.

Leonardo da Vinci famously wrote a one-page summary statement about health: how we should eat was on top of the list. Hippocrates, the father of medicine, believed that "all diseases start in the gut." Most cultures respect mealtimes, which historically have been honored and not rushed or shortened. The Chinese saying about drinking your food is another example of ancient cultures relying on wisdom to promote healthy habits. Many of our grandparents also respected mealtimes at the table and avoided talking while eating, focusing on chewing well. This traditional practice has been passed down from generation to generation for thousands of years.

Science and further reasoning.

If you eat slowly, you will likely eat less and lose weight. But if you eat too quickly and don't chew well, you will likely eat more and gain weight over time.

Multiple studies, including those by Harvard Health and Kyushu University in Japan, have shown the benefits of eating slowly.

They revealed that eating fast increases insulin levels and, as a result, insulin resistance and the development of metabolic syndrome, which is a risk factor for developing high blood pressure, HDL cholesterol deficiency, and weight gain.

Gastric bypass and stomach banding are surgical procedures that have been scientifically proven effective in sustaining weight loss and reducing the risk of type 2 diabetes, sleep apnea, cardiovascular events, and many other comorbidities. By limiting the amount of food and drink that can be swallowed at one time, the individual, after these procedures, has no choice but to eat and drink slowly, chewing well. You can achieve the same results without surgery. This is accomplished by practicing the habit of conscious eating—which I call *virtual gastric banding.*

Chewing food well, especially hard-to-digest foods like meat, reduces stomach acid and improves or cures heartburn and acid reflux. It also reduces the size of the stomach.

A distended stomach requires more food before the hunger sensation is gone. If we eat too quickly and don't chew well, then large chunks of solids will enter the digestive system and enlarge the stomach. The stomach doesn't have teeth, but it needs to break down the food we did not chew well. It does this by secreting acid. Unfortunately, this acid does not break down foods as efficiently as our teeth. For every extra ten to fifteen seconds of chewing, we may reduce the time food sits in the stomach by at least one hour. The prolonged digestion process, resulting from not chewing well, overfeeds the gut bacteria and can lead to *bacterial overgrowth*. Many recent studies, like the one published in the *British Medical Journal* in 2022, have linked our gut flora to obesity, type 2 diabetes, hypertension, depression, attention deficit disorder, chronic fatigue, irritable bowel syndrome, and more.

After finishing a meal, try to avoid sitting or lying down. Instead, stand up and walk for five to ten minutes minimum. This will allow the food to go farther down and reduce its accumulation in the upper digestive tract.

The nervous system has two distinct functional and structural components: the sympathetic and parasympathetic systems. The *sympathetic* system is primarily responsible for the body's interaction with the outside world, such as the fight-or-flight response. The *parasympathetic* system controls blood pressure, body temperature, digestion, and sleep.

Digestion is a predominantly parasympathetic process. Activities such as watching TV, reading, texting, and driving are sympathetic processes. The two systems alternate, oscillate and inhibit each other. When you are stressed, exposed to danger, or focused on a task, your sympathetic system becomes dominant, suppressing digestion and other parasympathetic activities.

Eating dinner properly improves sleep quality. Your sleep quality is reduced if you go to bed with a full stomach. Since your gut is still processing the food, the four sleep stages are disrupted for proper recovery. Inadequate chewing prolongs digestion, especially when eating later in the evening. If you eat dinner late, much of your night will be spent digesting the food, which should ideally be complete before you go to bed.

Poor chewing increases chronic inflammation in the gut and throughout the body. Eighty percent of your body's lymph nodes are concentrated around the intestines. One reason is that your gut can easily become like an open wound. Our body is more vulnerable in the gut because it needs to remain open to the environment to absorb nutrients. The gut is dirty and covered with trillions of organisms, bacteria, yeast, and viruses. These organisms outnumber the cells in the entire body. Most are friendly and protect the intestines from aggressive organisms that can invade through food. However, if the friendly organisms become disturbed—or if the unfriendly ones overgrow—then protection is lost. The immune system must then intervene by increasing inflammation locally and even generally.

Healthy gut flora is needed to digest food. Grinding food, chewing it well, and eating slowly to mix it with saliva are important in aiding digestion.

Eating your drinks means taking a sip at a time and drinking slowly. The concentration of minerals in water and other drinks is usually less than in our body fluids and blood. That is particularly true for the regular water that we drink nowadays, which is very poor in minerals. If we drink fast, that will create a sudden change in the concentration of minerals in the blood, as the absorption of fluids and water happens very quickly. The kidneys will get rid of some of the water by eliminating it fast unless we are dehydrated. There will be a shift of minerals also into the blood for the purpose of reducing the dilution. This will result in losing minerals and water. If we drink slowly, the body has time to adjust, and no significant mineral concentration shift will happen.

Eating your drinks is also essential for good digestion. This practice helps to bring the liquid's temperature closer to body temperature and mixes the drink well with saliva before swallowing. Gulping ice-cold drinks down can hurt your stomach. The stomach wall is thin and has much less blood supply than the mouth, so it cannot warm up as quickly. The entire drink, not just the sip, settles at the bottom of the stomach, and this causes cold-induced damage. Similarly, you should eat rather than drink smoothies or juices too. Mixing them with saliva is how the gut is designed to interact with their nutrients.

I have seen many patients cured of stomach discomfort and heartburn within a few days after practicing this method. They stopped drinking cold drinks or drank them slowly to allow the liquid to warm up before it reached the stomach.

I would like you to take from this chapter this: Learn how to slow down and chew your food and drinks well. You'd be surprised at how this simple change of behavior can significantly improve your health.

In summary:

Conscious eating involves eating slowly and chewing food well. It requires us to disconnect from other activities and induces a state of peace and meditation. It makes us eat less and still get better nutrient absorption. It has great benefits for digestion, helps us lose weight, and improves body inflammation.

Chapter 7

Meditating

Mind over matters, empowering the mind to heal the body and free the spirit.

"To think too much is a disease."

—Fyodor Dostoevsky.

Meditation has been practiced for thousands of years in various cultures and traditions and has been shown to have numerous benefits for mental and physical health. It is another constructive challenge for the restless minds we all developed as we were engulfed in the modern technological bubble. It can improve or even cure attention deficit disorders, anxiety, chronic tension headaches, migraine, insomnia, hypertension, obesity, and more. Indirectly addressing the above conditions will reduce the risk of cardiovascular disease, including heart attack and stroke, cancer, irritable bowel syndrome, and many other complications that can occur from the persistence of those conditions.

From the beginning, for thousands of years, the pace of life was far slower—until recent times. It became much faster, particularly after the invention of smartphones, when we started to multitask almost continuously as a habit. This sudden, significant change in our lifestyle goes against our design and is harmful. How often are you sitting down and eating without checking your phone? This continuous overstimulation burdens your brain and also wears on you physically and emotionally. It often leads to attention deficit disorders, which are becoming more common not only in younger people but even for those in their forties and fifties. The most vulnerable are kids under the age of ten.

Persistent overstimulation often leads to an addiction to adrenaline and other stress hormones created by chronic, repetitive stimulation. So, when things slow down, we'll go into relative withdrawal of stress hormones, which manifests in boredom and the urge to get stimulated again. It creates a strong intolerance to *stillness*.

Meditation is a practice that involves slowing down and focusing your attention on the present moment without judgment or distraction. It is a technique that aims to cultivate awareness in two main directions: inward toward your thoughts, emotions, and physical sensations as they arise in the present moment, and outward toward nature and your surroundings.

Let me ask you this: How long does it take for you to fall asleep at night? Does it take a while for your mind to shut off? If so, this is not surprising. Our pace of life is significantly faster even than twenty or thirty years ago, especially compared to the past few thousand years. Reaching this peaceful, relaxed, and disconnected state at night is now a challenge amid our fast and overstimulated world. Striving to adapt to this crazy pace, against our mind design, comes at a cost, making us physically and mentally ill.

This is why the slowing effect accompanying meditation is more important and effective now for modern man than ever.

Conscious eating is another form of meditation, described in depth in the Conscious Eating chapter. It will significantly improve your digestion, particularly helping with acid reflux, bacterial overgrowth, and obesity.

If we can learn to practice this type of stillness daily, we can return to our lives with a peaceful mindset. That is just one of the benefits of this type of meditation.

There are many methods of practicing meditation.

We can detach ourselves from the daily stresses and disconnect in many ways. Consider downloading meditation apps, such as Calm and Headspace. These can help you slow down as they help you look away from your worries and focus on your breathing instead. The purpose of this is to help you achieve perfect stillness.

Consider reading some books on the topic.

Next, I want to show you an example of outward-focus meditation toward nature and surroundings.

Here's a personal method type of meditation to start (to be used as a way to disconnect from routine, high-paced life):

Stand by the edge of a body of water—maybe on a beach, a lake, or a pool. Dip your feet into the water, and if possible, submerge your legs up to the knees. Stare out in the near distance, about a few feet ahead, and focus on the water. Observe the movement of different layers on the water's surface.

Please pay attention to every movement, noticing the various shapes, colors, and sizes of the waves and how they interact. Then, you may start to see patterns of movements beneath the water's surface. Watch how the light reflects from and penetrates the water. How do the air and the wind change these patterns?

Continue to observe and become more aware of these different types of patterns, both in the water's movement and the light's reflection. Now, without removing your gaze from the original area, expand your awareness of these movements and different intersecting patterns toward the periphery of your visual field. Doing this will shift and widen your focus until you fill the entire visual field with movement and changes. The more you embrace the sight, the more you will see. And the more you see, the more beautiful the sight becomes until you almost feel like merging with the water.

After practicing this exercise for a few minutes, you may experience this movement expanding within you, as if you have become part of the whole manifestation. Don't be surprised if you get overcome by a beautiful feeling of peace and awe. This practice allows your mind to become fully occupied with the hundreds and thousands of ever-changing movements sur-rounding you. This leaves no room in your mind for anything else.

In this way, we can explore the "space" of the small infinite realm while progressively increasing the number of details we perceive. Eventually, we may become lost in these details until the entire mind joyfully submerges and surrenders to infinity. This powerful and liberating experience will leave you in a serene state for several hours to follow. You may even notice that you become unaffected by the day's challenges and tribulations.

Since everything in nature is in a constant state of change and transformation, we can apply this same exercise of expand-ing awareness to different subjects in nature, such as the sky or trees.

At any time of the day, you can put activity on halt and focus on those smaller details of movements that occur around you—particularly in nature. Use your perceptions and senses to focus until you become completely absorbed in all the details. Not only will this allow you to unplug and disconnect from your surroundings completely, but this will leave you with no room to think.

Dealing with stressful thoughts.

We can deal with stressful thoughts that enter the mind in two ways. First, we can detach and become resilient, minimize impact, and learn to react to circumstances peacefully rather than with our natural, negative emotional reactions. Second, we can learn how to de-stress and disconnect from our daily lives by refocusing on a relaxing activity like exercise. These two approaches may intersect with each other at times. We could also try to avoid stressful situations, which can be challenging, considering that we can't always control life's circumstances.

I love this verse in the Bible that can pertain to the topic of de-stressing:

"Therefore, do not worry about tomorrow, for tomorrow will worry about itself. Each day has enough trouble of its own."
—Matthew 6:34.

If we hope to respond differently to the stresses of life, then there must be a shift in our values and expectations. How is this accomplished? Through both meditation and prayer. With these practices, we can move into the spiritual realm. And the more spiritual we become, our values—our treasures in life—will become untouchable, not threatened by the chaos of this world. That's because we transfer our values away from the horizontal level and place them on a vertical level.

The freedom to live in the present.

Thanks to our consciousness and developed frontal lobe, we are often too concerned about the future or react to the past instead of living in the present. The ancient Chinese philosopher and writer Lao Tzu said, "If you are depressed, you are living in the past. If you are anxious, you are living in the future. If you are at peace, you are living in the present."

Meditation is a habit and a powerful tool to live in the freedom of the present. The only true freedom is in the present because the past cannot be changed, and the future is mostly beyond our control. We all have certain degrees of post-traumatic stress, as naturally, we would like to avoid re-experiencing past painful experiences in the future.

It's human nature to attach ourselves to people and things in this world. But this can also cause suffering as we become dependent and vulnerable. We become weaker and more dependent by treasuring and attaching ourselves to things and people. These aspects of human nature and our relationship with God are addressed in detail in the later chapters.

This is why we must learn how to detach ourselves from this world. If we value our relationship with God more than with people or things, we will become stronger, more secure, and more stable. That is what this Scripture implies in 1 John 2:15-17:

"Do not love the world or anything in the world. If anyone loves the world, love for the Father is not in them. For everything in the world—the lust of the flesh, the lust of the eyes, and the pride of life—comes not from the Father but from the world. The world and its desires pass away, but whoever does the will of God lives forever."

Does this mean we should avoid loving and caring for people? Not at all! Rather, it means that we should aim to love and care unconditionally. In other words, without expecting to receive anything in return and without attaching ourselves to anything in this life. Doing this will enable us to become less vulnerable and enjoy more freedom in this temporary world.

As you can imagine, shifting our values this way goes against our natural impulses. This process requires regular, persistent efforts in the form of habitual prayer and meditation.

We can free ourselves from worldly attachments by entering stillness and practicing mind-emptying meditations. Then, we will have an enhanced ability to notice, appreciate, and connect deeper with God and His creation in nature.

I believe that God invites us to share the world, His beautiful creation, with us. He invites us to view our surroundings through a new lens and resonate with nature on a deep level.

You may ask: *Can I also connect with Him without thinking? Can I take in and admire the surroundings without allowing my mind to intervene in that moment?* Of course, you can. That, too, is a beautiful exercise. This type of awareness and observation is the most common source of inspiration for any artist and any art.

By practicing meditation and prayer regularly, our life's purpose can shift to focusing more on observing, understanding, and loving God and His creations. We can strive to act like Him by being creative, constructive, and serving and loving others rather than simply fighting against our abusive human nature. As we focus on growing into the first, we inevitably diminish the second.

Then, we will put this Scripture into practice:

"Therefore, I tell you, do not worry about your life, what you will eat or drink, or about your body, what you will wear. Is not life more than food and the body more than clothes? Look at the birds of the air; they do not sow or reap or store away in barns, and yet your heavenly Father feeds them. Are you not much more valuable than they? Can any one of you, by worrying, add a single hour to your life?"

—Matthew 6:25–34

Awareness of our day-to-day emotions, with purposely changing focus from negative thoughts and feelings to positive ones, is another important habit we should practice. You can read more about that in Chapter 10: The Habit of Checking the Emotional Sign and the Initial Drive.

I hope you are encouraged to recognize your ability to transform your mind. Instead of your mind being a source of stress, it can become a source of health, peace, and inspiration.

In summary:

Meditation implies slowing down our minds and increasing awareness. It involves either complete disconnecting and mind emptying or focusing on a particular subject. It helps us detach from the past or the future and live in the present. Meditation helps reduce the symptoms of anxiety, depression, and attention deficit disorders.

Chapter 8

Praying

Starting and cultivating an honest and personal relationship with God.

"Praying is asking God to relate to you on your terms but in His strength."

—Pastor Mark Batterson

Praying is the act of communicating with a higher power or deity through words, thoughts, or actions. It is a form of spiritual practice often associated with religion and involves expressing gratitude, asking for guidance, forgiveness, or help, and seeking comfort or support. Prayers can be performed in various ways, including reciting memorized texts, reading sacred texts, or silently meditating.

It is in our nature, almost as a need, to hope and believe. But it certainly matters to consider the object of our hopes and how we relate to it.

Praying implies believing in someone or something so powerful and sovereign that we cannot entirely comprehend.

Through prayer, we achieve important things:

We relieve inner tension and conflict by accepting and transferring control to the higher entity. This allows us to attain peace and rest through humility, repentance, and acceptance of our limitations.

If we pray habitually, we develop a relationship with God, which will significantly help us grow wiser and become stronger.

As we grow spiritually, we will relate better with our peers and be able to help others in need.

Praying should be habitual rather than as needed.

I recommend a habitual lifestyle of prayer, as the Bible says: "Pray without ceasing" (1 Thessalonians 5:17). Many people tend to only pray on a particular occasion, when there is a need, or when they are suffering (or their loved ones). And that's okay. But if we hope to receive the full benefits of an authentic relationship with a far superior and intelligent being, we must pray regularly with different motives.

James 1:6 says, "But if any of you lacks wisdom, let them ask of God, who gives to all people generously and without reproach, and it will be given to them."

Habitual prayer should be mostly private, as it involves a personal, direct relationship with God (or whoever you consider the Creator and the entity in control.)

Matthew 6:7 says, "But when you pray, go into your room, close the door, and pray to your Father, who is unseen."

When we pray, let us first begin with an attitude of gratefulness. We can be grateful for what we have and the mere fact that we can pray and relate with God. We can be thankful for the opportunity to walk if we have all our limbs. We can be thankful for the opportunity to think. We can even be thankful that we are capable of appreciating what we have!

We tend to want less when we appreciate and remain grateful for what we have. This can help us to be more content, joyful, and happy.

God *wants* to relate with us. Yet, we are more likely to run to Him when we suffer. It's in those moments that we run back to Him. His comfort during those times prompts us to remain with Him.

Unfortunately, our modern culture allows little room for God. Instead, this materialistic culture tempts us to have many other idols. These idols keep us blind and will ultimately lead to suffering.

Regular praying involves accountability and compliance.

When we pray regularly, we will continue to grow into the person we were designed to become. We become spiritually stronger. That's because communing with God involves developing a relationship with Him. In this relationship, we are not just asking and receiving—because, as in any healthy relationship, we should *also give*. We must be honest, accountable, and responsible and avoid asking about things we can accomplish for ourselves. For a relationship to function in a healthy manner, each party must have common interests and work to expand them.

We should know what God wants from us. And if we hope for and expect His help to arrive, then we must show Him that we are devoted to following His will. We know He would be pleased and proud of us when we follow His Word.

We could pray, for example, for safety in those split seconds when we change songs on the car stereo or answer a text while driving, a momentary distraction that could easily result in a serious accident. We hope for protection when we are vulnerable, like each time we briefly divert our attention from the road, an action we all do hundreds of times a month.

As we become more assertive in our special relationship with God, we become stronger and more efficient in all our relations with the people around us. We learn to care for, give to, and forgive others.

"Who comforts us in all our troubles, so that we can comfort those in any trouble with the comfort we ourselves receive from God" (2 Corinthians 1:4).

As this relationship evolves through prayer, meditation, and spiritual practices, we will learn to see the world through God's eyes. We will disconnect from our temporary, insignificant daily life with its routines and worries. Gaining His perspective helps us to see where His values lie. This enables us to fulfill our higher purposes as we become more and more like Him.

"Consider it pure joy, my brothers and sisters, whenever you face trials of many kinds because you know that the testing of your faith produces perseverance. Let perseverance finish its work so that you may be mature and complete, not lacking anything" (James 1:2-4).

So, as we grow, our object of praying continues to change as well. It changes from being exempted from certain sufferings to accepting and even *appreciating* the challenges. In the long run, these challenges will make us stronger.

If our prayers remain unanswered, we must strengthen our trust and accept that we will be rewarded in eternity, even if we suffer in the short term.

Either way, we can trust that God cares about us so much that He hears our every prayer to Him. *"I have told you these things so that in me you may have peace. In this world, you will have trouble. But take heart! I have overcome the world"* (John 16:33).

In summary:

Praying is a means of connecting and relating with God. It is a way of acknowledging that we do not have complete control over our lives and putting our trust in a higher power. Prayer helps us to deal better with difficulties and conflicts as it encourages us to hope. It is a great source of peace and stress relief as we express gratitude for what we have and surrender control.

Chapter 9

Napping

Disconnect, reset, and recover in just a few minutes.

Napping, or taking a short sleep during the day, can reap great results for both physical and mental well-being. Napping may last from as short as thirty seconds up to one hour. Sometimes, a short nap lasting only a few minutes can do as much good as a few hours of regular sleep.

Here are some of the most notable benefits of napping:

Increased alertness and productivity: This is especially true for people who may feel tired or drowsy during the day. A brief nap can boost energy levels and improve focus, increasing productivity and performance. If you regularly have significant fatigue and daytime sleepiness and snore while sleeping, consider taking a sleep test. This will determine whether or not you have sleep apnea. Although sleep apnea is mainly related to obesity, that's not always the case. If a case of sleep apnea goes untreated, in moderate to severe forms, it can lead to multiple health issues and may shorten one's lifespan. Besides, decreasing the quality of life can also increase the risk of heart attack or stroke. A sleep study can be conducted with home kits or in a sleep lab. Talk to your primary care physician if this is a concern for you.

Improved mood: Napping can help improve mood and reduce irritability, frustration, and stress. It can promote feelings of both relaxation and rejuvenation.

Improved cognitive function: Napping can help improve cognitive function. This includes memory, learning, and problem-solving abilities. It can also help enhance creativity and promote mental clarity. A lack of sleep can negatively interfere with your learning efforts if you are studying or trying to learn something new.

Reduced risk of accidents and errors: Napping can help reduce the risk of accidents and errors, especially for people who work in safety-sensitive professions or who operate heavy machinery.

Why is sleep so important? Because sleep deprivation is extremely harmful to our bodies, especially if it becomes chronic. The quality of sleep is almost as important as the *quantity.* Many studies prove that night shift workers have an increased risk of cardiovascular events and shorter lifespans. The fact that sleep deprivation is sometimes used as a form of torture shows us just how vital sleep is for life.

Do you want to improve the quality of your sleep? If so, there are some simple measures you can begin to implement daily.

First, try to go to bed at the same consistent time each day—ideally before 11 p.m. Remember that our ancestors did not have electricity, so they had little choice but to go to bed just after the sun went down. We are still genetically pre-designed by our ancestors' way of life. Therefore, try to avoid eating late as well. It's ideal to avoid eating at least three to four hours before bedtime.

It is also recommended to minimize the amount of alcohol you consume with dinner, as this can interfere with sleep quality. This is especially true if you consume more than one glass of wine or beer.

Remember that most sleeping pills and sedatives prolong sleep, but with a significantly reduced quality. Ideally, we should dream at night. If you do not have dreams, consider taking a sleep study to rule out sleep apnea and other sleep disorders.

Many books have been written about sleep. These books dive deep into discussing sleep architecture, sleep hygiene, and how we can naturally improve sleep and help people with chronic insomnia. We need to try to fix the root cause of all sleeping problems. Despite advancing technology, we still don't know much about sleep and dreaming, but their vital role in maintaining optimal health is clearly understood.

Most animals nap easily and frequently. If you have a pet, you're well aware of this. This is because they live in the moment. Not all of us can nap easily. That's because we rarely live in the moment and are almost always wired. Worrying about tomorrow and other concerns keeps us in a state of tension. This is extremely unhealthy, especially if this becomes a consistent and prolonged habit.

Unfortunately, the pace of our lives is much higher today than fifty years ago. Our genetics are not designed to handle this high pace frequently. As mentioned previously, this pace of life has been increased by the overstimulation we receive from smartphones and other advanced technologies, as well as our tendencies to multitask. This has made it more difficult for us to nap but has also made it much more critical. Your body needs a break. So don't feel guilty about giving yourself this downtime. You can do this by napping, meditating, exercising, or simply relaxing by listening to music or enjoying the outdoors.

Here's my method for falling asleep (at night or during the day): I like to concentrate on an imaginary, beautiful scenario that brings me to a calm state. For example, this could be an imaginary scenic hike I envision for an upcoming trip. Or I can imagine that I am taking pictures of a unique moonrise or at the opening reception for my new art gallery. Whatever the imagined scenario, this will help to disconnect me from the day's overwhelming stimulation and project me into a pleasant, carefree state—and it's in this state that I soon fall asleep.

Napping involves two essential conditions. First, you must listen to your body. When you feel tired, you must avoid resisting the urge to rest and instead give in. You don't need to be very tired to nap.

Second, you must disconnect from daily stresses to shut down the mind. This will also make it easier to focus on a pleasant and relaxing thought.

Ideally, a person should nap in bed since napping in an unphysiological position can result in injuries—particularly neck pain. But you don't need to have a bed to nap. Just make sure your sleep position will not result in a strained neck or a numb arm. If you can sleep in the plane or the car without any issues, you can apply the same position technique for napping during your work breaks. Sometimes I will nap at work using a travel pillow—on my desk, in my office chair, between late patients, or at lunchtime. Three to five minutes is all I need.

It's ideal to avoid taking naps later in the day, such as after 5 p.m. Doing so may interfere with your regular night sleep patterns.

It is best to wake up from naps in the lighter non-REM (rapid eye movement) sleep stages, such as stage one or two, or during the transition between non-REM and REM sleep cycles. You can do this by keeping the nap short. Doing this can help you feel more refreshed and alert upon waking up.

It is generally not recommended to wake up during the REM sleep phase—the phase where most dreaming occurs. Doing so can disrupt your natural sleep cycle and leave you groggy, disoriented, and tired throughout the day. This is why it's best to try and keep the nap duration shorter than one hour—so you can avoid going into the REM stage of sleep.

At night, you cycle through several non-REM and REM sleep stages. Non-REM sleep is divided into three stages, with the deepest stage being the most restorative for the body. REM sleep typically occurs ninety minutes after falling asleep and happens several times throughout the night, with each REM phase lengthening.

We cannot overestimate the importance of sleep. Besides the immediate negative consequences described above, persistent long-term lack of sleep will make us age faster and increase the risk of dementia, vascular disease, and even death.

In summary:

Napping refers to sleeping for a short period, ranging from a few minutes to one hour. The need for napping should not be resisted, as it often suggests that we are not getting enough rest at night. In such cases, it is crucial to take measures to ensure a good-quality night's sleep. However, if obtaining a good night's sleep is not possible, it needs to be investigated further to rule out sleep apnea or other sleep disturbances. Persisting improper sleep or reduced sleep leads to serious health consequences like an increased risk of heart attack, stroke, and Alzheimer's disease. Poor quality of sleep also results in poor recovery from daily stress and reduced life quality and length.

Chapter 10

The Habit of Checking Your Emotional Sign and Initial Drive

"Neither pleasure nor pain should enter as motives when one must do what must be done."

—Julius Evola

If we were facing each other right now and I asked how you were doing, how would you respond? You might respond as usual: "I'm fine; how are you?" And yet, how many times have we given that answer while masking our distress with a smile?

It's important, however, for us to become aware of how we truly feel on a routine basis. How we actually feel will likely fall into one of three categories: positive, negative, or indifferent. We can learn to become aware of our feelings by regularly checking and identifying our emotional signs. More of this later, below.

The source of the initial drive.

We must learn to recognize if our feelings are the initial triggers of our actions.

Why is this important?

First, let's consider the choices we make daily. Many of these everyday decisions result from an interaction between emotions and thoughts, feelings, and mind. This is mostly an unconscious interaction. But we need to consider this: What prompts us to make these decisions? The cause of choice is known as the initial drive or the *trigger*. And this trigger is born in either the mind or the feelings. Which one?

Sometimes, it's difficult to discern which came first, the idea or the feeling. For example, suppose you must choose to donate to one of the two candidates for your political party. Most of your friends prefer one of them because they know the candidate personally, and the candidate is more charismatic. The other candidate is older but has a history of proving that he keeps his word and can implement the policy promised. If you choose the first candidate, you most likely follow an emotional drive as you like charisma, don't want to upset your friends, and you need to avoid peer pressure. Choosing the second candidate follows a good principle, and your feelings will adjust to accept and align with the principle.

Jeremiah 17:9 says, "The heart is deceitful above all things and desperately wicked: who can know it?" That statement is very accurate. Our emotions can often lead us down destructive paths. That's why, when making important life-changing decisions, the mind should be led by a constructive idea, not by primitive instincts and emotions.

To help us with this, we should become self-aware. We must develop the ability to discern our original main drive in any important situation. Self-awareness requires us to ask ourselves if we are driven by our ideas and principles or our primitive drives.

Romantic relationships teach us a great deal about the importance of being self-aware. Stable, *agape* love is born in the will, whereas "falling in love" or romantic love (*eros* in Greek) is emotionally driven. *Agape* or unconditional love can make you dislike and criticize someone you love, as those may be the appropriate attitudes for the higher good for the other person. You align your emotions to the will as you follow the noble idea of wanting and doing the best for someone (which can involve disagreement and conflict).

Agape love in its pure form does not expect reciprocity. It does not expect anything in return. It is unconditional. On the other hand, erotic or *eros* love fades if the other person does not share the same feelings and is not strong enough to go against the other's wishes. Unfortunately, relationships based merely on romantic love do not usually last.

To illustrate this *agape* love, several years ago, my parents encouraged me to leave them in Romania and go to the United States, even though they needed me. I am their only child, and they did not have a lot of support. Many of our relatives have passed away, and the others live too far away. My parents' love for me superseded their desire for me to live close to them. This is *agape* love.

So, when we make decisions, what initiates our thoughts? Is it the will to follow a principle—or are we mostly led by our needs and emotions?

We have the privilege of being able to recognize which drive prompted a decision. And we have the power to choose to follow either ideas or feelings.

Apostle Paul describes this battle between the heart and mind in Romans 7:18: *"The Conflicts of Two Natures: for the willing is present in me, but the doing of the good is not. For the good that I want, I do not do, but I practice the very evil that I do not want."*

We are emotional beings.

When an idea drives us first, unavoidably, our emotions will attach and align to this idea, sooner rather than later. We naturally associate our primitive drives, emotions, and needs with new ideas. Still, it's important to remember that the mind and the emotion are a two-way connection, and we can recognize which one came first and the predominant direction of action.

The direction should flow from the idea to the will. Then, from the will to the mind—and, finally, to the emotions. Ideally, this direction should not be reversed, but it will always travel in both directions. Back and forth. It is natural for a drive to travel from emotions to the will. Only when we practice awareness can we make the right direction predominant.

We cannot live without emotions, but we *can* transform and redirect them. A pure state of mind is rare—for example, when making calculations or studying for a test; a purely emotional state is more natural—for instance, when listening to music.

However, the most frequent state we find ourselves in is one where the mind and the emotions coexist. Since the mind can manipulate our feelings, it is more powerful than emotions—but it can only briefly operate independently of emotions. This is human nature.

It is typical in everyday life for conflicting drives and emotions to attempt to interfere and change the direction of influence.

Suppose your mind and your will move together in a direction opposite to your emotions' direction. In that case, to sustain the will and succeed, you will need to attach a new emotion to it that follows your will's direction against the initial feelings.

For example, if a colleague is angry at you and attacks you verbally, you naturally respond with anger and defensiveness. You'd become reactive with similar negative emotions. On the other hand, if you become aware that he is actually suffering on the inside and dealing with frustration and negative emotions, then you may develop compassion instead of reactive anger. You may be more willing to try and understand the other person, even if they are not right. That is an example of a *mind-driven* choice followed by a *positive* feeling—compassion.

It's all too easy to adopt an idea that originates—mainly, if not entirely—in our emotions and primitive drives. Just consider the growing number of tattoos and piercings teenagers and young adults are getting now. Many choose tattoos and piercings because it is a trend or they admire someone with tattoos, so they believe they'd look good with them, too. And looking good brings positive emotion and satisfies them.

Some people come to God by heart, and others come to Him by reasoning. Then, the mind may align with the heart or vice versa. If we don't have good, reliable principles, we will end up with all kinds of sects and cults. These have exploded for the past few generations due to a lack of culture, mental discipline, and respect for ancient wisdom.

It's important for the heart to align with the mind-driven principles. We cannot last long if the two go in different directions or ignore each other. You cannot go far if you don't put your heart into what you do. On the other hand, if you follow the heart alone, you will likely end up lost, astray, and most likely not in a good place.

We most often open up to God when we are suffering. It helps us relieve stress. But without suffering, loss, or other significant events, we often fail to relate with God, especially if we are driven by the heart. We should change this, open up to Him, and remain grateful.

Most of the time, we are driven by primitive emotional needs that dominate the background like a continuous noise. "I don't like that it's hot outside … I'm worried that I'll run out of gas … I'm annoyed that I have to make dinner … I'm anxious about my parents."

Now that we understand these concepts, how can we apply them?

Our natural inclination to attach to the negative and the importance of redirecting it into the positive.

As mentioned in the beginning, we can assign a sign to our feelings and emotions at any moment. And most often, we will have two choices—a positive choice or a negative one.

Are we joyful, optimistic, relaxed … or angry, anxious, upset, or pessimistic?

It is important to realize when we get stuck in the negative. It's our nature to blow things out of proportion because whatever we focus on may greatly expand beyond reality. Are we focusing on the empty half of the glass or the full half? It's our choice. Emotionally, we tend to choose the empty part. That is also instinctual, as unfavorable may be associated with a threat, and threats awaken survival instincts. But the will and the mind have the power to choose the other way.

We need to make a conscious effort and make the better choice. Let's expand the full part of the glass by focusing on that instead. We should materialize the choice into action. The action that supports the positive view will help us to keep the focus in the right direction. Suppose you're upset about something and don't feel like going out with friends. If you meet with them anyway, it will usually help you take your focus away from the negative feelings. We can almost always find actions that make us follow the will in a positive direction and improve our mood.

Isn't knowing that we have control in this area a relief? It is within our power to check in on our emotional state daily by checking our feelings regularly. This is especially significant when we make important decisions. Then, we must recognize when we are stuck in a negative mood and refocus—preferably through action—and change that negative state into a positive one.

We can also track the origin of our intentions and actions. We should initiate necessary actions (based on acceptable principles or ideas) rather than becoming driven by an emotional need. We need to ensure that we do not get tricked by rationalization and falsely believe that the *mind* was the trigger when, in reality, *feelings* came first—as happens often.

Good is constructive; bad is destructive.

How do we define a good or bad principle or idea? That is an essential and tricky concept to grasp. Simply put, *good* includes the constructive and the creative; *bad* includes the destructive and the chaotic. From another perspective, *bad* is what often causes us to suffer unnecessarily. *Good* is the opposite. It grants us joy, peace, love, and so on. For a believer in God, it is easier: bad is everything that goes against God's will, and good is what fulfills God's will.

Sometimes, though, it's not so obvious, or even impossible, to define what is destructive versus what is *constructive* or where God stands. One of the main purposes of this book is to define and clarify what is good and what is wrong from a broad perspective.

If the initial drive, the trigger of our actions, originates in a good principle and we experience positive feelings, we will evolve into a constructive state—toward stability, peace, and order.

Yes, having positive emotions is good, but following them against good principles is not good. If a spouse falls in love with a colleague at work, dwells on it, and becomes obsessed, that is destructive for the marriage and for their children's lives.

Following negative feelings and wrong principles, we will end up damaged and in chaos.

Following good principles with adverse emotions cannot get you too far, especially in the long term. It is unsustainable to have persistent negative feelings, even if we follow a good principle.

For example, if you decide to swim in the ocean as a regular workout but fear sharks, then that would be hard to sustain. You may adjust and swim in a pool, find another cardio workout, or somehow resolve the fear.

On the other hand, if it is a temporary situation and doesn't need persistence, following the will and good principles should bring you to a better place. Even if it is painful and embarrassing, speaking the truth is almost always the right thing to do.

Certain situations can be complicated and complex, so there may be some exceptions to these rules. But they are rare.

Most healthy constructive habits involve stepping out of our comfort zones. They demand discipline and persistence. In the past, we faced these challenges regularly, not because we chose to but because life was tough. Today, however, we must take them on voluntarily, following healthy, good principles, which makes the task more difficult. Yet, we have the privilege of doing so at our discretion. To sustain long-term challenges that we undertake willingly rather than being forced into them, we require good understanding, motivation, and a robust, well-organized system. In the next chapter, I will provide you with another tool that will help you sustain healthy habits.

In summary:

It will be highly beneficial to develop an awareness habit that checks our emotional state on an hourly basis. This should also establish the role of our emotions in triggering our more relevant decisions and actions. Living in a persisting negative emotional state is detrimental to our physical, mental, and spiritual health. Using good principles as initial drives for our decisions and actions and aligning our emotions with them would be the solution and the desired way of living. Successfully handling our emotions to prevent them from causing harm requires a solid understanding of human nature and ancient wisdom. More detailed information about these issues is available in the later chapters of the book.

Chapter 11

Measuring and Trading Discomfort and Suffering

"We must all suffer from one of two pains: the pain of discipline or the pain of regret. The difference is discipline weighs ounces while regret weighs tons."

—Jim Rohn, motivational speaker

The trouble with immediate gratification.

One of our most significant issues is choosing delayed pleasure over instant gratification. Even though ancient wisdom and modern science demonstrate that deferred satisfaction brings multiple rewards regarding our well-being, we consistently opt for the easier option. We choose to fulfill an immediate impulse.

An interesting illustration comes from a Stanford University study, which found that children who chose to wait to get two marshmallows instead of accepting one straight away were more likely to succeed in later life.

When we intend to change habits, it's essential to consider that our nature and genetic makeup will persuade us to indulge in immediate gratification at the expense of delayed gratification. More often than we realize, we practice immediate gratification. Our nature makes it difficult for us to think objectively about what will happen in the near future, let alone try and understand something further down the line. Nonetheless, each decision has consequences—some rapid, some postponed, some visible, and some insignificant.

"He is the most powerful who and has power over himself."
—Seneca, Roman philosopher

Abstaining from snacking on cookies when you're hungry requires effort, and it can be uncomfortable—but giving into this temptation continually over time can lead to more significant discomfort in the form of fatigue, weight gain, sugar cravings, and more. Let's consider our gratification actions as a trade-off for long-term benefits. Sure, getting up early to exercise might be challenging at the moment, but you'll feel energized and gain mental clarity soon after—plus, you'll see overall health benefits down the line. Remember: what may seem distant now will one day become immediately relevant.

Controlling our immediate impulses can sometimes be critical. For example, if we receive a text while driving, answering the message could result in the loss of human life. This is why self-discipline is a necessary trait for us to master. If we can train ourselves to practice self-discipline in one situation, that will soon carry over to other facets of our lives.

"That which is escaped now is pain to come."
—Traditional proverb

Units of hardship.

Consider immediate versus postponed gratification or the coin flip: discomfort now versus discomfort later. Theoretically, it may be simpler to identify, comprehend, and manage our present impulses if we calculate the discomfort involved in "hardship units." Enduring a difficulty, whatever the kind, prompts a physiological rise in stress hormones like adrenaline and cortisol, a surge in pulse rate, and an increase in muscle strain. These changes represent the associated physical and mental stress.

I define one hardship unit, or one HU, approximately representing a similar increase of the above combined physiological changes over a limited period, like one minute, by an average of ten percent. Let's also say that one HU results from the temporary discomfort of a healthy habit—such as skipping a meal during intermittent fasting, waking up earlier for exercise, taking the stairs at work instead of the elevator, or admitting a mistake at work to your boss.

One HU also results from fatigue, the inability to sleep for some hours, or having a moderate headache or backache. This is all relative and may vary from person to person; however, this hypothetical perspective on hardship will allow us to better understand and compare discomfort and suffering. So now let's fast forward five to ten or fifteen years into the future. How many more units of hardship do we experience due to an unhealthy lifestyle in our past?

In addition to these delayed and hard-to-revert, remote consequences, there are also more immediate, temporary consequences, usually experienced on the same day or week. For example, ending your shower in cold water for two minutes will give you good energy and mental clarity right away, lasting for many hours. That will cost you, let's say, one HU, as it is intense but short. The reverse, ending the morning shower with hot water, will make you more sluggish and less alert for a while. That will cost you at least the same discomfort because even if it is not that intense, it lasts a lot longer. Here, the perception is misguiding because the acute, intense discomfort is a lot more obvious than the slow, longer-lasting fatigue. Of course, there are all the long-term great health benefits of cold plunges described above.

There is an old truism that reinforces the value of resisting unhealthy impulses:

"An ounce of prevention is worth a pound of cure."

Hardship is unavoidable. Let's learn to trade hardship units.

A great trade-off occurs when we consciously reduce the total amount of HUs over time. We have two choices: first, we can follow a healthy (yet often uncomfortable) route by exercising regularly, eating nutritious meals, getting enough sleep each night. Let's say these account for sixty HUs per month or two per day. Our second option includes opting for instant gratification and skipping discomfort, leading, sooner or later, to health issues, including weight gain, back pain, anxiety, fatigue, etcetera. All these resulting symptoms are accumulating many more HUs, as they are persistent, even if they are more easily tolerated.

Further down the line, it may cause more serious conditions such as diabetes, heart attack, or cancer. If we choose the second option, within two years, we may suffer ten times more with hundreds of HUs per month. Not to mention that there are significant, measurable financial gains by being disciplined and staying healthy.

"It is easier to resist at the beginning than at the end." According to Leonardo da Vinci, preventing yourself from straying down the wrong path is easier when you're just starting instead of later. The farther you go down the wrong road, the bigger the leap you must make to switch to the correct path.

Voluntary, immediate discomfort is usually more intense and acute, yet shorter-lived, whereas the delayed, consequential hardship (that results from unhealthy habits) tends to be less intense but lasting and often permanent. As the damage builds up bit by bit, it produces mild or subtle symptoms that our body gets used to. Being developed so slowly, the damages are escaping our awareness of their presence until it's too late; this is often the case with cancer or vascular disease. Being overweight or having high blood pressure or sugar levels may not hurt initially as they develop insidiously.

We can't separate suffering associated with unhealthy habits from suffering caused by emotional states—sadness, anger, stress. Of course, there are events in life that are outside of our control, such as accidents or losing a loved one. But there is a lot of suffering that we *can* avoid or at least reduce. How? We must recognize and trade immediate HUs for delayed and remote HUs. We must become savvy traders!

We acquire knowledge about trading through our own experience or that of others. If we're adept learners, we can save ourselves a lot of grief, particularly by following in the footsteps of others. Though it may not come naturally, we must fight our instincts and rely on the experiences of others instead of our own.

> *"The only way to keep your health is to eat what you don't want, drink what you don't like, and do what you'd rather not."*
>
> —Mark Twain

In summary:

You need to look at the big picture and understand that the way nature is, it makes discomfort and suffering unavoidable. But not all pains are the same, you do have a choice. You can choose voluntary discomfort now in exchange for a lot more suffering later. Be a smart trader.

You may have realized by now that our biggest obstacle to long-term success in applying constructive principles is yourself.

To conquer yourself, you need to first understand yourself very well. In the next chapter, I'll provide insight into exactly what in your nature is damaging to your well-being.

Chapter 12

Understanding Human Nature

The troubles with the conscious mind.

Would you consider human nature to be essentially bad? I certainly do. Because somehow, no matter what, we tend to cause ourselves and those around us much unnecessary suffering.

How is that possible?

I'll tell you how: The conscious mind is to blame. It allows us to abuse what we like or want. The conscious mind can easily push us to extremes.

Technical evolution adds even more to this by significantly expanding our options.

In our search for pleasure, comfort, and control, we end up causing much damage.

As it is our nature to abuse what we like, we must learn to discipline, control, and practice moderation.

Of course, we also face plenty of unavoidable suffering from life challenges. These often provide learning and growth opportunities.

We need help limiting our propensity toward damage and redirecting us toward good outcomes. The help comes in the form of spiritual wisdom and knowledge from modern science.

Do pain and other negative consequences follow all pleasures? Not at all. We can find joy, fun, and pleasure in the direction of the higher purpose that often comes with pain-free consequences—learning and applying new skills, creating, and sharing art, playing sports, and other competitions.

It is not the selfishness but its direction that matters.

Each of us desires to achieve based on our own values, and there are two crucial questions we must confront:

1. What values do we embrace?
2. Does our personal gain directly or indirectly contribute to the gain or the harm of others?

Furthermore, we must consider whether the gains others receive from us align with our values or theirs. Even an act of genuine sacrifice, like a mother willingly giving up everything, including her life, for her children, is still rooted in self-interest. She simply places a higher value on her children than on herself. We should not deny that we are always driven by self-interest and the pursuit of personal gain. Selfishness is inherent in our nature—it is natural. However, the difference lies in whether we include others in our self-interest or only focus on ourselves.

In the Bible, God calls upon us to include others, especially Himself, who represents the greatest and highest value. Doing so assures our gain—not always in this earthly life, but certainly in eternity. Therefore, we need to understand what our Creator desires from us and then act accordingly.

If we accept the idea that a vastly superior being has created us, it becomes logical to seek understanding regarding our purpose for existence. We should strive to comprehend why we were created and with what intention. Subsequently, it would be wise for us to embrace that purpose wholeheartedly. (I discuss this complex issue in detail in the final four chapters of the book.)

The new challenges of our modern times.

Most known knowledge and wisdom on human nature have already been discovered as far back as 3,000 years ago. King Solomon wrote, "There is nothing new under the sun" (Ecclesiastes 1:9). What is new is only the *form* and the *context*, not the essence. Yet even though human nature hasn't changed much since ancient times, advancements in technology and modern science have dramatically changed our way of life— especially during the past one hundred years. We are highly creative and inventive. These traits are integrated into our very nature.

In addition, modern times offer us many options, possibilities, and temptations. This means that, in many ways, it is more challenging to live a good and healthy life today than in the past. This also means that following protective health rules and habits is more imperative than ever before. We are offered far more opportunities today than our ancestors ever had. A middle-class Westerner today has many more options and possibilities than a king had two hundred years ago.

We must watch carefully what we get involved in. The types of pleasure we engage in create the kind of suffering we will experience.

For example, drinking excessively often leads to alcoholism. This, of course, can affect everyone connected with the alcoholic. In the long term, we know alcoholism leads to much unnecessary pain.

Sadly, we are often too preoccupied with pleasure and fun—so much so that we usually don't pay enough attention to principles and virtues. We want to gain in the direction of our hope. We place hope in what we believe has value and will grant us purpose.

But we often place value on the wrong things. The new cultural bubble we are being engulfed in is the biggest culprit.

Take Hollywood, for example—along with the entertainment culture overall. The rate of disasters and crises is relatively high among celebrities and those who have reached a high level of success. Drug and alcohol abuse, divorce, and suicide are prevalent among the famous. Just think about the many celebrities we have lost in recent years due to these issues. This should remind us that true happiness and peace are not synonymous with attaining everything you could ever ask for.

Protecting us from ourselves.

Many great thinkers have taken up the issue of human suffering throughout the ages.

Buddha, for instance, was raised in luxury, yet he left his family and lived in the woods. He spent many years in solitude, meditating on ways to reduce human suffering and minimize human nature's negative impact on self and others. Much of the Christian Bible is focused on human nature as well. One of Jesus's primary purposes in his ministry was to help reduce humanity's suffering, at the individual level.

Today, modern writers and philosophers join the ancients to address the issue of self-inflicted human suffering. Jordan Peterson, author of *12 Rules for Life*, is a great example, along with Scott Peck, who wrote *The Road Less Traveled* and Daniel Gilbert, author of *Stumbling on Happiness*. Thousands of books exist on this subject.

Some great thinkers have developed clear and practical concepts that have lessened suffering over hundreds and thousands of years. These concepts have aided in civilization's advancement. Many are found in the scriptures and founding texts of the main widespread religions and the U.S. Constitution. Notice how most of these texts address human nature and protect us from self-harm at the social level.

Many laws and regulations already protect citizens and limit the damage we inflict upon other individuals. The issue remains: How do we protect the individual from himself? Spirituality addresses that question well, but science provides far fewer principles and rules of self-governance.

What follows are the main characteristics of our inner nature that often make us vulnerable and prone to damage and suffering. Consider how we relate to the statements below:

1. We project and attach emotions and primitive drives to ideas and things.

Our primitive instincts' manifestations—such as fear, pride, and lust—are not limited to helping our survival. We also attach them to ideas. We project, associate, and attach ourselves to tangible items and beliefs. For example, have you ever "suffered" profoundly when your favorite football team lost the Super Bowl? Maybe you can relate to that emotion, even if your feelings concern something unrelated to sports.

Sometimes, we confuse an idea with a survival threat, mostly subconsciously. Fueled by fear, greed, pride, or lust, we become blind and prepared to fight and even die for an idea. Animals cannot do this because they do not have beliefs. History shows that humans often developed ideologies that proved to be extremely blindfolding and dangerous.

In the name of an *idea*, we can become blind and can even transform into a monster.

Think about some incident when you had a hard time admitting you were wrong. Here's why that happens: Once we align our drives—like pride or fear—to an idea, it is hard to change our minds and detach based on reasoning—even if the idea is later proven wrong. We become blind. Changing our minds may even feel like an existential threat.

In the United States, the division between Democrats and Republicans in recent years illustrates projection, association, and attachment to ideas. Political associations often break up businesses, friendships, and marriages on a large scale. Many attach to an ideology created by contemporary culture, often not even realizing it.

If we take a glance back into history, we will see this same lesson. Humans have committed suicide and genocide after believing a particular idea—it is the power of our mind that manipulates our drives and emotions to such an extent. As a great Romanian philosopher, Emile Cioran, said:

> *"Ideas should be neutral. But man animates them with his passions and folly. Impure and turned into beliefs, they take on the appearance of reality."*

Stalin, Mao, and Hitler are just a few examples of men who, following their ideologies, caused mass suffering in our recent history. Terrorists and suicide bombers are killing themselves for an idea, overriding their most powerful instinct—the survival instinct.

The idea is the most potent drive for change that man will ever encounter.

Attaching our primitive drives to ideas has also caused racism, anti-Semitism, and all other forms of selective discrimination to exist. We tend to identify with groups with interests, cultures, looks, and values similar to ours. We feel distant and even threatened by our differences from other groups. This is due to our basic primitive survival instincts. We can also witness this amongst animals at a more basic level.

But nowadays, we should not merely survive or allow primal drives to lead us.

On the other hand, attaching positive emotions to constructive ideas can result in *good*. In sports, as well as in science and technology, we keep breaking record after record. Runners are prime examples. Many track athletes train vigorously and regularly to become fast enough to break new records. For the average person, numerous community races raise funds for various causes in competitions for runners of all ages. Many times, competition fuels progress.

2. We fail to anticipate and foresee real consequences.

Another harmful characteristic of human nature is that we regularly fail to foresee the future accurately. In fact, we are far from that, even with respect to the near future.

As a result, in our continuous search for comfort and gratification, we are more likely to choose *immediate* rather than *delayed gratification*.

Immediate gratification is a major issue.

Sometimes, we ignore the mere fact that *consequences are inevitable*. We want to believe otherwise. This is why we sometimes intentionally choose to "forget" the consequences of overeating. But if we keep up that harmful habit daily, the consequences will likely catch up with us eventually.

If we overeat, we gain weight. If we continue, we can become ill with type 2 diabetes or high blood pressure. But for some reason, as we stand in front of an open pantry or refrigerator in search of a snack or leftover cake, we easily make ourselves believe that it will not hurt us. We give in because we think we are exempted from harm this time.

But the thing is that "one time" is hardly ever just a one-time event because the same thing happens again the next day and then the day after that.

Unfortunately, we often don't have a wake-up call until we receive an unfavorable diagnosis. Only then do we realize that change is necessary.

Why do we so easily believe that *what happens to others will not happen to us?*

It is because of our huge capacity to ignore—as the saying goes, "Ignorance is bliss." *We ignore it because we need comfort.* So, the only way to avoid this is to discipline ourselves, not automatically follow the easy way. Comfort should be seen as potentially dangerous, and we will fail less by practicing good habits that make us comfortable with the uncomfortable.

Is it impossible for us to overcome our desires for satisfaction, comfort, and control? Of course not. The question is, how else can we endure discomfort without caving under its pressure?

One other answer is *fear*—the fear of consequences. But we often like to believe that there are no consequences. And that is when we usually fail.

"We all make choices, but in the end, our choices make us."
—Ken Levine, American video game designer, creative
director, and writer

Though human brains, compared with those of animals, have a well-developed frontal lobe that is the center of planning, foreseeing, and preventing, we often repeatedly fail to predict the future correctly. Sometimes, our shortsightedness and our consistent practice of immediate gratification come with significant repercussions. In other words, our old primitive limbic system—responsible for basic impulse to win in the battle with the newer developed frontal lobe.

Even if there are immediate consequences, we fool ourselves about them—for instance, we can convince ourselves that drinking heavily and driving is okay. "Just this time … it will be fine …" And yet, tens of thousands of car accidents and deaths happen every year in the United States alone because of drinking and driving.

The antidote to immediate gratification.

Now that we understand our tendency to dismiss consequences, how can we protect ourselves from making this mistake?

First, we have to self-train to recognize and understand when and why we give in to immediate gratification.

Then, instead, we should find comfort in the positive results of delayed gratifications. At the same time, we should push our awareness and become afraid of the negative consequences of giving in.

For example, if someone cuts you off while driving, your impulse is probably to react angrily, right? And yet we know that reacting in this primitive way, as an immediate gratification choice, could increase the risk of serious injuries. So, instead, you can become aware of your bruised ego and decide to remain non-reactive and in control of your impulses.

Even more efficient than this is to train yourself to implement a replacement habit that will interfere and stop the often-habitual process of immediate gratification.

Healthy habits are immensely powerful tools that can counteract immediate impulses and needs. They enable us to "do what is meaningful and not what is expedient," as Jordan Peterson explains in his latest book. Good habits give us stability and structure, and they can keep us from falling prey to chaotic, primitive driving influences.

If we become hungry after eating an early dinner, for instance, we have choices. We can develop a habit of drinking water with minerals and staying away from the kitchen. We could (and should) stop buying snacks, too. These habits can make a big difference in our health in the long term. It requires discipline.

"Discipline is choosing between what you want now and what you want most."

—Abraham Lincoln

This is what it looks like to strengthen our will by developing a corresponding *proper* habit. A habit that can replace the original (more) primitive impulse.

Natural selection acts with full power and kills the "weaker" ones even today—just as it did in the jungle thousands of years ago. Only today, natural selection occurs quite often because of our bad habits, which are becoming the new/modern dangers, part of the new cultural bubble we are all getting engulfed in. Just think of texting and driving and how that, among other careless behaviors, can influence the more impulsive and less disciplined among us. These behaviors can also have a devastating impact on the innocent.

One simple good habit can save many lives. The habit of resisting the immediate gratification impulse … like resisting the urge to check a text message while driving, or resisting the urge to change lanes without looking for other vehicles.

"While we are free to choose our actions, we are not free to choose the consequences of our actions."

—Stephen R. Covey, American educator and author

The danger of high or wrong expectations.

Unrealistic anticipations create yet another unwanted setup. We often develop unreasonable expectations. These lofty expectations set us up for disappointment and unhappiness. All this is self-inflicted and completely unnecessary.

This self-inflicted harm happens because there is a massive gap between what we can imagine and what we can *do*. Animals do not have a conscious mind, so they have more limited imagination and abilities. We have the freedom to imagine almost anything without limits, but we only seldom have the power to achieve it.

We fail to see marriage as an important, necessary challenge in life and as the building block of societies from the beginning of civilization. We get married with totally different expectations, particularly in modern culture. Marriage, according to the old wisdom, is not equivalent to mere romance, convenience, and comfort. It is a commitment. For a healthy marriage to thrive, couples must sacrifice their own interests for the common good. It is an act of will, liability, and accountability. It fulfills a higher purpose.

Modern technology can worsen the reality gap.

Furthermore, thanks to advanced technology, we can practically live in a virtual world. This further increases the reality gap between what we imagine and what we can do. When we sit behind a screen and can choose and even control what we see, we become unchallenged and thus could easily become radicalized. Consider what Facebook and other social media platforms have enabled us to do. We often limit our exposure to like-minded groups and groups that think the same way we do.

The advancing technology and science of modern times, by increasing the diversity of options and range of possibilities, greatly increases the differences between people, individuals, and social classes. New technology gives more people access to success, increasing the chances of reaching maximum potential—yet it's also increased the number of options, including bad choices and temptations, leading to unsuccess and failures.

Confusing needing with wanting.

A lot of stress comes from the conflict or tension between what we want and what we can have or do. This was a lot less in the past as the options were reduced. Before the modern technological advances of the 20th century, the tension was mainly between what we need and what we can have, as we had a much more difficult life. Today, we often have everything we need, but we end up confusing what we want and what we need. That's a source of significant unnecessary suffering. We see evidence of the harm caused by virtual environments in teens' mental states today. The increasing amount of time that teens spend in a virtual environment corresponds with a growing rate of teen depression and suicide. Social media has only amplified destructive human behavior. Since there are fewer rules and limits than in real life, there are also fewer apparent and fewer immediate consequences. Social media is so new that we have not had the time to figure out how to protect ourselves from something so different from classic and typical dangers. Furthermore, our actions on social media often disregard the same principles that ancient wisdom cautioned us to heed regarding human nature.

Can morality stop us and motivate us to respond appropriately?

Many times, the answer is *no*. Morality can be tricked, subverted, and manipulated through rationalization or other ways.

In the early 2000s, how we listened to and purchased music was transformed. Millions of people switched from listening to music on CD players to mp3 players and iPods. This meant that people no longer purchased CDs at music stores; instead, they downloaded music from iTunes or other sources.

It didn't take long for millions to bypass paying for these songs, so billions of songs became downloaded for "free," despite being illegal. Why did so many people commit this unlawful act? Because they rationalized that not buying the song was not considered stealing. Yes, technically, it was theft. But there were no consequences. So ... why not?

Another harmful characteristic of human nature is that we regularly fail to accurately foresee the future, as explained above. In fact, we are far from that, even for the near future.

As a result, in our continuous search for comfort and gratification, we are more likely to choose *immediate* rather than *delayed gratification*.

3. We live in a primarily reactive state.

How many times have you tried to pass someone, and the slower car suddenly accelerates? The driver can be tempted to react in the same way, as it can be contagious. But doing that will easily provoke a similar response from the other person and may trigger some dangerous road rage. This is an example of the primitive drive operating in pride or envy. They are powerful and, unfortunately, most of the time destructive.

You see, since we are social animals, we are reactive beings. We often do things and act impulsively, driven by the behavior or emotions of others.

In a dialog, an aggressive, raised tone of voice can easily provoke a similar response from the other person and may trigger a serious argument.

Do you remember the shortage of toilet paper during COVID-19? In mid-March 2020, the world went crazy buying rolls of toilet paper—so much so that stores and even manufacturers ran out. Why did this happen? As mentioned above, behaviors, thoughts, and emotions can be contagious, as we are so easily reactive. It is called herd behavior.

We have all faced some degree of post-traumatic stress.

Studies have shown that we are happier and live longer when surrounded by friends and loved ones. When we're isolated, we often struggle and suffer. Conflicts and challenges are natural occurrences in human society. And for the younger and most vulnerable, these challenges can lead to persistent feelings of shame or guilt. These are common reasons that keep us isolated as well. This especially applies to kids and adolescents.

Being isolated can also make us more vulnerable and reactive later in life. We wrongly value the things that protect us from these negative emotions.

A kid, for instance, may prefer to stay "safe" at home and connect through social media with other peers rather than meet them in person. An adult may prefer to stay single or work at a less-desired job instead of facing a new challenge.

We did not have these "protective" choices a few decades ago. Nowadays, however, with the new comfort culture, we have become more intolerant of conflict, uncertainty, risk, and change. So, we lose the capability to adapt, be flexible, and even to be grateful. Challenges help us grow and make us stronger and humbler.

No matter what life experiences we've had, we have all experienced some degree of post-traumatic stress disorder (PTSD). It makes us reactive to anything connected with past traumatic events—consciously, yes, but mostly *subconsciously*. We learn to cope with it most of the time. If we become aware (conscious) of these past hurtful experiences and their connection with the current experiences—and if we clarify our emotional reactions—we will be able to improve or resolve our responses. Some will need therapy to uncover the origin of the issues and learn to handle them better.

To do this, though, we must become courageous and determined, especially for those already affected functionally. If we shift values from the ones that make us comfortable to the ones that make us better and stronger, progress will begin to occur. Shifting values requires both motivation and belief. And *that* requires proper knowledge, reasoning, and understanding.

> *"The secret of change is to focus all of your energy not on fighting the old but on building the new."*
>
> —Socrates

Uncovering the initial drive or conflict.

Marsh Rosenberg, a doctor in psychology, has a principle of nonviolent communication that offers a concrete solution to the above problem and involves following a principle. It consists of following the mind to discover the emotional drives behind what makes us do what we do. We can change the way we satisfy our needs and feelings by discovering them as being at the root of some of our more hostile actions, which at first seem unrelated. Because inner emotional conflict is part of nature and basic survival, aggression is often expected to be the prominent leader in our actions.

The solution here is to identify your own feelings and inner conflicts and have the courage to present them as being the cause of your actions rather than just stating or criticizing the actions.

Suppose, for instance, that one of your friends behaved inappropriately in front of your family. Instead of criticizing the behavior itself, you would just express to the friend the way it made you feel, such as feeling embarrassed, ashamed, or guilty.

Using wisdom, sound principles, and a leading mind over emotion, we can clarify and uncover these conflicts and let the basic needs and feelings be revealed so we can express and fulfill them in a nonviolent, non-aggressive, less conflictual way.

When we can see the root of our actions, it is easier to have compassion and understanding for others and ourselves. This requires an educated awareness. It can make a difference in choosing the way to satisfy our needs. We will be able to avoid complicated, convoluted actions and means. We will be capable of relating directly and clearly and less conflictually.

Instead of lashing out during a couple's argument, nonviolent communication involves identifying and expressing emotional needs in a non-threatening way, which can help reduce conflict and improve relationships. For instance, saying, "I feel neglected and unloved when we don't spend time together," is better than accusing the other of not doing what you would like. This takes courage as we will open up and admit our vulnerability.

> *"When you react, you let others control you. When you respond, you are in control."*
> —Bohdi Sanders, American author, martial artist, and
> motivational speaker

4. We naturally have a strong temptation for more and different.

The Roman philosopher Seneca wrote, *"It is not the man who has too little, but the man who craves more, that is poor."*

Although this was written before AD 65, his words remain true today and offer a glimpse into another element of our destructive nature.

How many times have we claimed to have nothing to wear when our closet was filled with clothes? The desire to have more—or to desire what we do not have—can become never-ending.

Why do you think technology companies continue developing new updates and models yearly? Because they rely on human nature's tendency to desire something new and different. Once a year or so, these companies release new models for their smartphones, TVs, cameras, cars, on so on.

Social media certainly doesn't help us control our thirst for more. It only serves to exploit this thirst within us even more. Why do you think it's programmed to detect our interests? So it can feed us more about what we are looking for. In the process, it only worsens this addiction of ours.

Consider, for example, American families' average credit card debt today. We've gotten into the habit of buying items we cannot afford, expecting we will easily pay for them in the future or over time. Again, the consequences of our actions are far from our minds when we create habits like these.

The comparison effect.

I enjoyed watching movies on a small thirty-inch TV when I was young. But over time, what happened? Larger models became available. So, TV watchers quickly traded their old models in for a fifty-inch TV screen.

What if, after enjoying the newer model for some time, we returned to the smaller model? We would be unhappy and even struggle with the backward change.

You see, it all comes down to *comparison*. Because what happens after we get too accustomed to that fifty-inch model? Soon, we will have a desire for an *even larger* TV. The excitement we once had over that fifty-inch model has been forgotten. This is what Theodore Roosevelt meant when he said, "Comparison is the thief of joy."

Comparison is one of the essential functions of life. Essentially, it is the basis of information. So, everything is based on comparison. Without comparison, there is no data. The most primitive life form uses comparison to perform any task. That's because comparison is the flip side of change. It concerns every living level—from the bacteria that measure the change of the protein concentrations in an environment to the Wall Street money market that measures changes in stock value, or our body receptors that measure the difference in temperature between skin and the environment.

There is no survival without comparison. It's the only way to perceive change, and we cannot avoid or escape it.

Many of us frequently live in a cyclical or roller-coaster pattern. We first become aware, then have a desire, and then act to achieve it. Once we enjoy fulfillment, we often abuse it. Then, we have post-fulfillment melancholy, become bored, and repeat. This can happen with eating, sex, shopping, vacationing, and so many other activities. While the object of desire may remain the same for a while, we eventually grow bored and want to change that as well.

"Eat to live, not live to eat."

—Socrates (469-399 BC)

Unfortunately, the vast majority of films and television shows today seem to rely more and more on elements like violence, murder, sex, deceit, or significant crime to maintain our interest. If they fail to tap into our primal instincts, our attention and interest tend to wane. Without the appropriate cultural exposure and education, it becomes challenging to appreciate and be engaged in nuanced, more sophisticated, nonviolent themes and concepts. As we become desensitized to these dramatic themes over time, increasingly extreme and unrealistic plotlines are introduced to keep us entertained. What disastrous sources of education and inspiration do the new generations have?

The love–hate paradox of change.

It's interesting to see how paradoxical and contradictory our human nature is. Yes, we frequently and consciously look for something new, different, and more. Yet, at the same time, we subconsciously desire routine. We develop an attachment to things and often fear change. This contradiction can create much drama within us. Our desire for something *new* and *different* is why we tend not to appreciate what we have until after we've lost it.

While we need and attach to the familiar, we are still curious and interested in new things. Curiosity is a powerful instinct, even in animals. That's because curiosity emerged with survival instinct. We desire to *know*, and it quickly becomes a need to *know and understand*. Knowing gives us both comfort and security. And this, in turn, produces control or certainty. Control and assurance would provide us with a better chance of survival.

The power of diversity.

Did you realize that even animals choose diversity over survival? That's because the need for diversity comprises part of their nature.

An experiment was conducted to prove this. A mouse chose mating with a new female partner in heat rather than essential food and water—to its death. The variable in this experiment was the "new partner" factor because the mouse stopped mating with the first new partner and chose to eat after a while. However, if a new female were introduced repetitively, the male would not stop. This experiment is seldom possible in real life. Humans, however, may easily create a similar situation.

This can help explain one reason why divorce rates are so high. In our modern society, people have become more driven by their primitive drives than by their morality and principles.

Last year, my wife and I traveled to Italy. On this trip, we visited a few Catholic churches—I was surprised to discover that my wife was forbidden to enter it. Her shoulders were not covered.

As I considered this, I realized that most major religions worldwide have traditionally required women to dress modestly, to cover their shoulders and knees, or be completely covered in public—in some major religions, even today. But many reformed churches are also to blame, as they permit improper dressing in the name of freedom. Look at how most women are dressed in a lot of non-denominational churches. Men's average clothing didn't change much over time, but the way most women dress today is extremely different from even fifty years ago.

Knowing very well the weaknesses of human nature, these traditional religions intended to minimize distractions and men's temptation to view women in a sexual way and for women to take advantage of it.

Modern cultures are often just the opposite, especially in our Western civilization. It's sad to see so many women and teenage girls dress and behave like sexual objects, inviting lust. It seems impossible to avoid this. We're exposed to this on TV, in movies, on social media, and out in public, even in churches.

I would claim this to be one of the main reasons relationships nowadays are brief and unsteady. It is a significant factor in the high divorce rate.

This also explains the success of the porn industry and why it continues to expand. This industry is also very damaging. Many studies and statistics support this statement. According to the National Coalition for the Protection of Children & Families, 47% of families in the United States reported that pornography was a problem in their homes. Pornography use increases the marital infidelity rate by more than 300%.

As I mentioned, the type of pleasure we seek defines the consequential pain we encounter sooner or later.

Properly handling our primitive drives.

Pleasure, fun, and joy don't need to be followed by suffering and pain. It is the *abuse* of sources of pleasure that can have negative consequences. It's okay to enjoy these activities—yet we must enjoy them in moderation. We must know how much is *too* much and remain self-aware. Yes, this means that we need to discipline ourselves. It is because of our inherited nature that we almost always want more. We get bored quickly and end up abusing ourselves and others.

It is in our nature to compare ourselves and our situations to others. We do this with food, sex, money, power, and control. We are driven by powerful primitive instincts like survival and reproduction, with undesirable manifestations like lust, pride, envy, and greed. This can constantly interfere with our intentions and actions.

Yet when we create something constructive or beautiful— or get involved in arts—we can have fun and experience joy without the risk of painful consequences. That's because being creative almost always aligns with the higher purposes. It often involves connecting with nature and with God.

The routine and the adrenaline.

If you haven't noticed it already, we are addictive human beings.

One of the worst forms of addiction is our universal addiction to our own adrenaline levels. Once we've repeatedly experienced sustained high adrenaline states, we may become addicted to this. When the adrenaline high wears off and we experience a lower level of adrenaline, we may feel unfulfilled.

This is why, once we taste the joy of high-speed downhill skiing (without being overwhelmingly scared of falling), we want to do it again and again. *Speed* and *danger* create that high adrenaline state that makes us feel more alive because of the risk. We often become addicted to taking risks—or rather, we become addicted to the adrenaline accompanying the risk. And, of course, here also intervenes the other drive discussed above. The wanting for *more*. This happens consciously or subconsciously. This is how we become thrilled by adventures. Even procrastination can become a form of addiction to adrenaline. Once an activity becomes repetitive and part of our habitual routine, we often lose interest.

For instance, can you recall the very first time that you drove a car or stepped into a new home you bought? Imagine what it would be like to experience that same thrill of newness each time you drove or came home.

The good thing is that the older we become, the more we appreciate what we have. But we also become pickier and harder to impress or please. We become less tolerant and less flexible. That's why we tend to need more routine as we age.

Interestingly, we can also become bored more easily by things we make than those in nature. I never grow tired of seeing the sky or the ocean. Of all human creations, art is usually the most entertaining. Again, this suggests that we have a strong attraction toward diversity and change. I elaborate on this concept in Chapter 16.

Much damage comes from our inability to cope with mandatory routines.

Many of us face difficulty managing compulsory routines, especially at work, which can often lead to significant issues. If we fail to form an emotional bond or cultivate an active interest in our responsibilities, we risk becoming disengaged, akin to malfunctioning robots. This disconnection from our duties can foster apathy and lack of motivation, resulting in diminished output quality and potential errors. One remedy for this natural propensity towards inattention and disinterest lies in cultivating discipline and awareness of consequences. The problem is that it is not our nature to put someone else before ourselves.

However, it's important to acknowledge that while discipline and routine can be effective aids, they cannot fully compensate for the lack of passion and genuine care. Maintaining consistent interest, care, and, most importantly, passion over extended periods can be challenging. The quality of service can fluctuate greatly depending on how these factors are addressed and structured within a company's policies.

To illustrate this, consider the service reputations of the United Parcel Service (UPS) and the United States Postal Service (USPS). Generally, private enterprises considerably outperform governmental counterparts, mainly due to the two factors mentioned earlier. Private companies often benefit from more refined operational protocols and superior policies to motivate and reward their employees. Employees in these private enterprises often have more "skin in the game." Government employees usually suffer little or no consequences if they underperform.

The same comparison can be made on a national level when evaluating governments and private entities. A comparison can be drawn between the United States and several Eastern European countries—analogous to UPS (the U.S.) and USPS (these other countries). In these Eastern European nations, the communist and socialist policies have vastly diminished individual self-interest and private ownership in favor of collective societal benefits.

5. *Whatever we focus on expands.*

We have an amazing capacity to see only what we are looking for, which can blind us to inconvenient truths. We must remember the principle that whatever we focus on expands and becomes more significant, sometimes pushing us further away from the truth.

Consider the processes of falling in love or idolizing a celebrity. Both examples involve an inclination toward selective attention and augmentation. A vicious cycle mechanism can be found here—because the more familiar we are, the more attracted and comfortable we become with a favorable situation, person, or object. Social media currently exploits this as well.

Imagine if a Republican were to become a Democrat or vice versa. While this can happen, it's certainly not a common occurrence. It would also be extraordinary if an atheist became a Christian or vice versa—if based on theoretical arguments alone.

Philosopher and psychoanalyst Carl Jung said, *"Ideas have people, not the other way around."* This is how ideologies are consolidated.

How do panic attacks manifest? Following a traumatic trigger, a panic attack is typically prompted when our "focus" becomes deformed, and that aspect of reality becomes amplified in our minds. When we hyper-focus on a particular threat, it becomes subjectively much more significant than it is in reality; that's when we can become thrown into a panic attack. In the brain, it corresponds to a functional and even structural formation of fast-beaten paths of neurons that fire easier and quicker. These paths are formed through repetitive use as a result of amplified and persistent focus.

The power of placebo.

The placebo effect also shows how subjective, reactive, and easily influenced we can become. In many drug studies, the placebo is as effective and even more effective as the real thing.

The placebo effect can be stronger or weaker depending on its presentation. For example, let's consider the placebo effect of sham acupuncture. Fake acupuncture was applied for this in a study published in *The Journal of Headache and Pain*, where it was used to treat headaches. The placebo was enhanced by contextual factors, including elaborate treatment rituals, higher levels of attention, and physical contact. This is to be compared with oral pharmacologic placebos, proven to be much weaker, in which the subjects were just told that one of the pills is the real medicine while the other is a sugar or placebo pill, and they will not know which one they are having. These results tell us different degrees of response to placebo treatments depending on how elaborate and significant they become for us.

We also widely differ in how we *respond* to placebos and what we choose to see.

It is a simple choice but still a hard, deep-rooted one.

The choice we make—whether to focus on the glass half-empty or half-full—makes a big difference for our psyche. If we can see a situation from the half-full perspective, we can become full of courage, optimism, and hope. On the other hand, if we focus on the half-empty glass, we can become discontented, angry, depressed, and anxious.

The reason we choose one half over the other is rooted in our *subconscious*. Often, we choose to reinforce a familiar state, which could be either optimism and hope—or fear, anxiety, and pessimism. Our subconscious searches for and chooses a familiar state based on prior experiences and habits.

The survival instinct and the need for comfort and security drive these choices. Our minds then follow the drive and start to elaborate, rationalize, and justify these decisions. If we experienced prolonged states of negative emotions in our formative years—such as fear, guilt, or shame—then sadly, we may become comfortable and familiar with regularly dwelling in those states. We may subconsciously look for them, especially in stressful situations. That's because these familiar negative emotions paradoxically provide the impression of stability and security.

It's a natural human tendency to concentrate on negative aspects of our lives because they often represent potential threats. These threats command our attention because they challenge our survival, either directly or indirectly.

For example, consider a typical evening: you might find yourself lying in bed, preoccupied with worry about a potential conflict at work the next morning, such as a disagreement over vacation schedules that could lead to your plane ticket being canceled. This concern overshadows the positive event you have planned for later the following day, a delightful dinner with old friends visiting from out of town. This pattern occurs because our minds are wired to prioritize potential dangers to ensure our survival, even in situations where the stakes are not life-threatening.

Most people prefer to avoid the challenge of the new, un-known, and uncharted path. There is also a significant genetic predisposition and capacity for tolerating uncertainty and change. This applies to the propensity for optimism or pessi-mism as well.

Anais Nin's famous quote aptly explains why we amplify situations from either a negative or positive perspective: *"We don't see things as they are; we see things as we are."* Distortion of reality is a common and natural habit for us humans. Many of the fears we develop have more to do with our weaknesses and insecurities rather than actual threats. Suppose a person suffers from an unrealistic fear of drowning every time it rains—even if a flood warning is not a real threat. The reason for this fear is not based on reality; instead, it could be rooted in a traumatic experience and often an inability to swim.

6. We often choose to learn from our own mistakes instead of the mistakes, experience, or wisdom of others.

Many times, we do not learn from our own either.

Our inner nature's intelligence urges us to learn from our experiences. This stems from our survival and adaptation process. This primitive mechanism is inalterable in animals. However, as beings with a conscious mind, we can do better and learn from the experiences of others, or even worse, we can ignore our own past experiences that we could have learned from.

Unfortunately, it is unnatural for a man to act upon a simple new idea that does not directly or immediately involve a strong primitive impulse like fear, pride, or greed. Most of the time we need stronger motivations to react unless we discipline and educate ourselves to follow principles.

> *"To make no mistakes is not in the power of man; but from their errors and mistakes the wise and good learn wisdom for the future."*
>
> —Plutarch

Consider how you learned the skills and education needed for a job or profession. You accepted and followed the rules you were given, right? These rules were based on the experience and knowledge of others in the field—those experts who have gone before you.

The same cannot be said about our private and social lives. How we live our private and social lives depends on the culture around us. Not long ago, personal aspects of life were taught in school and at home to a greater extent than they are today. However, nowadays, social media play a more significant role in cultural behaviors—even more so than our home and family influences. This isn't just true among our younger generations. It's true for most of us.

If we learned and adopted certain valuable principles—such as keeping family first or respecting and helping our parents— we would be protected from much unnecessary suffering. And yet we often, as a society, disregard history and our ancestors' wisdom. Interestingly, each generation tends to repeat the same mistakes. We often refuse to learn from the mistakes of those before us.

"By three methods we may learn wisdom: First, by reflection, which is noblest; Second, by imitation, which is easiest; and third by experience, which is the bitterest."

—Confucius

One solution could involve implementing human nature awareness classes in schools at various levels. These classes should be nonpolitical and focus on subjects like: Delayed Gratification, Embracing Discomfort, Self-Discipline, Non-judgmental Thinking, Willpower over Impulses, and more. These programs should include theoretical and practical components to facilitate a comprehensive understanding.

Additionally, mandatory world history and geography classes and basic economic and financial education should be introduced in middle and high school. Presently, most high school and even college graduates possess limited cultural knowledge and perspectives, making them vulnerable to cultural manipulation, indoctrination, and radicalization. By broadening their understanding of the world and equipping them with essential multidisciplinary literacy, we can empower students to think critically, make informed decisions, and resist manipulation.

With these educational initiatives, we can promote self-awareness, critical thinking, and resilience among students. This holistic approach aims to enhance their development, protect them from negative influences, and foster a more informed and discerning generation. We can stop this new cultural bubble from engulfing, brainwashing, and poisoning us.

7. *We are too quick to judge.*

Humans tend to judge too much and too often. Our natural inclination is to judge the person instead of just the facts. This often leads us to develop wrong conclusions, see through a distorted reality, and find ourselves in conflicts. This subconscious, vicious cycle happens to anybody who is not careful about avoiding this distortion.

Once we become aware of a fact, we may quickly jump to a conclusion without enough information and verification. The reality is almost always more complicated than we can comprehend initially. Then, we quickly simplify and align our emotions with that idea. Or perhaps we were emotionally ready, and the idea only supports and fits our need or mood to criticize or control. Then, we begin to rationalize and find new facts and information to align with our emotions. But these emotions now become amplified, and so the cycle is perpetuated.

Misunderstandings based on texting behavior are common, whether they relate to delayed responses, messages that come across as inappropriate, or other issues. However, it's crucial to consider that technical issues can often influence how messages are received or sent. Before forming conclusions about someone's intentions, we should remember that our perception of their texts might not fully capture their true intentions. Taking a moment to consider these possibilities can help avoid unnecessary conflicts and misunderstandings. When we judge public figures, it is even easier to be wrong as the information we usually have access to is incomplete and often altered or manipulated. Nevertheless, it ends with significant polarization of opinions.

These situations show how quick judgments can lead to incorrect conclusions, distorted reality, conflicts, and misunderstandings.

The more knowledgeable and intelligent we are, the more tempted to judge we become.

For those like me, a follower of Christ, we must remember this biblical advice found in Matthew 7:1, *"Do not judge…"*

This is where intelligence and wisdom go in opposite directions, as wisdom has a broader perspective.

"To attain knowledge, add things every day. To attain wisdom, remove things every day."

—Lao Tzu

Intelligence without wisdom is dangerous.

When we cast judgment on someone, we often act as though we are in a superior position. This gives us a false impression of control over that person. It satisfies our primitive survival instinct. We need both humility and compassion to prevent that from happening. When we judge others, we also risk becoming emotionally overcharged. It's easy to hold a grudge against someone who bruised our ego. Sure, that person may have been in the wrong. Still, when we continue to dwell on the issue, we become emotionally recharged repeatedly in a negative manner.

This advice goes hand in hand with another important source of suffering, in the following section.

8. We don't know how, and we don't want to forgive.

Forgiveness goes against morality because morality asks for both fairness and justice while forgiveness does not. It implies strength, as it requires relinquishing our pride. Forgiveness terminates unnecessary suffering on both sides and provides immense relief of tension and pain for both sides. When we forgive somebody, we often forgive ourselves at the same time.

When we judge too quickly and refuse to forgive someone, we may later find ourselves dealing with discontentment, anger, anxiety, depression, insomnia, and all the physical manifestations induced by these prolonged sufferings. That's because this kind of judgment and unforgiveness are the root cause of these issues. The Bible is very clear on this issue:

"Love prospers when a fault is forgiven, but dwelling on it separates close friends."

—Proverbs 17:9

"But I say to you who hear: love your enemies, do good to those who hate you."

—Luke 6:27

The family is the main pillar of any prosperous society. In the new Western culture, it is in great danger.

All aspects of human nature described above also represent serious challenges for keeping a family together.

Besides amplifying the destructive effect of our own nature, the new culture creates new, even more harmful threats to the stability of the family and society. Advanced technology creates multiple powerful, novel, destructive temptations. It exploits our natural propensity to look for more and different, to abuse what we like, and to become bored with repetition.

Whether we are shopping online or in a mall, we are exposed to young women provocatively dressed or almost naked in ad images or in real life while shopping. Then you see a newer, better version of your phone or TV. And then you see the unlimited variety of clothing and shoes, some very different, some similar to yours but newer.

Moreover, the new culture went further and not only brought the right of women and race or ethnic minorities to vote and have the same social status, which is great but also made them compete and go into conflict with those not like them.

Today, women are encouraged to compete with men for job positions and other roles in society. That goes against nature's intelligent design, which made males and females very different for survival and constructive purposes. Women and men have been designed to take different roles in family and society, which are complementary, not competing. In today's culture, in the name of equality and non-discrimination, as women are encouraged to compete with men at the same time, they still must be mothers and take care of their children. This creates a lot of tension in society in general and inside the family in particular. It leads to a decreased number of children, an increased divorce rate, and an aging population. It also shifted the average age of marriage later in life and significantly increased the number of singles and single parents.

For a stable, beautiful relationship between a husband and a wife, we must understand our primitive, destructive nature and follow a disciplined will. The will should be led by good, constructive principles rooted in wisdom and spirituality, not by the new brainwashing modern propaganda.

For a marital relationship to last, there should be a combination of each of the following important ingredients: friendship, playfulness, respect, and good sex. They are necessary to counteract our primitive, destructive inclinations:

- Friendship to counteract or balance our reactive state nature and our propensity to judge and not to forgive.
- Playfulness to help us deal with the inclination to get bored and not to forgive.
- Respect to help us appreciate and learn from others' wisdom and experience and judge less.
- Good sex to satisfy our needs for more and different and to learn to forgive.

In summary:

The more we understand and manage our human nature, which has remained relatively unchanged since ancient times, the more likely we are to attain complete and genuine well-being. Sadly, our new modern culture further exploits and amplifies our weaknesses. A toxic bubble has been forming in Western civilization, and it is expanding into other cultures. This also threatens the very foundation of our society: the family unit. Ancient wisdom's way of handling our nature is the solution. Adopting our ancestors' values and learning from their mistakes rather than our own would save us from a lot of unnecessary suffering. There are many good books that address these issues.

All these human flaws are unavoidable, and dealing with them affects us not only emotionally or mentally but also physically, with the potential to damage our health and well-being. In the next chapter, I address the issues with modern Western medicine in the 21st-century toxic culture.

Chapter 13

Modern Medicine in the 21st Century

"Health is a state of complete physical, mental, and social well-being, and not merely the absence of disease or infirmity."

—Hippocrates

Brian, a young patient in his mid-20s, has been under my care for at least five years. Until recently, he had been relatively healthy, experiencing only occasional heartburn and increased abdominal bloating. However, a couple of years ago, he came to my office with new symptoms of painless rectal bleeding and a moderate exacerbation of his digestive problems. He also complained of new-onset muscle cramps that were becoming more persistent and debilitating. Lately, Brian had been experiencing more stress and had been neglecting his diet, consuming more processed foods high in carbs.

I put him on an aggressive lifestyle change regimen that included eliminating unhealthy foods, adding intermittent fasting, and stress-reducing measures. He underwent extensive workups, including blood tests, allergy tests, colonoscopy, and upper endoscopy, which showed only nonspecific inflammation in the colon and moderate gastritis. All other tests came back negative. Although Brian's heartburn symptoms and muscle cramps improved after implementing lifestyle changes, such as increasing hydration with mineral water and shifting to a mostly carnivore diet, the bleeding did not improve much.

After six months, he discovered that he had an adverse reaction to one of the components in the coconut oil he used to put in his coffee. Once he stopped consuming it, the bleeding stopped as well.

I also diagnosed Brian with stress-induced irritable bowel syndrome, as his digestive symptoms would flare up with stress and poor diet. A genetic test showed that he has a double MTHFR gene deficiency, which I treated with increasing fermented foods in his diet and intermittent use of 5-L methyl folate and B12 supplements, with some success. When Brian strictly follows the recommended lifestyle changes, he feels much better.

What is causing so many problems with our well-being? What makes us sick? How can we get better?

In this chapter, I present a simplified and clarified perspective of the main issues that make us unhealthy, the causes, and the solutions. This will improve your expectations and the way you will handle your health.

After finishing this chapter, you will be able to recognize, understand, and apply concepts such as these:

- Chronic, underlying, disease-predisposing factors versus triggers
- Aligning your lifestyle to your design
- Breaking hidden vicious circles and creating positive circles
- How to demand and get from your inner resources healing and well-being

We face health issues from two principal sources: internal genetic elements and external assaults.

We have two main external access points, open portals, where we are generally defenseless and where the assailants habitually enter our body: one point is the mouth, and the other is the mind.

Whatever we put into our mouths cannot simply be discarded. We must process it, assimilate it, and only after that use, deposit, or eliminate it.

Similarly, whatever we expose our minds to cannot be erased and leaves a more or less profound effect on our psyche and emotions.

When the food we consume produces waste or stress in our body, it turns into aggression. The body often reacts with inflammation or is thrown out of balance, causing harm. The more processed the food, the more likely it is to produce waste.

Similarly, whatever we allow into our minds can't simply be wiped out. If it brings on uneasiness or distress, it often becomes harmful if it persists or is intense.

Recently, a new fragile portal into our body has become increasingly significant—and that is our airways and lungs. What we breathe in from the air and environment becomes more important as air contamination has been rising in the past few decades.

We all have different susceptibilities to these aggressors, some of which are pre-determined by our genetics. We have the capacity to recover, but this can be hindered by two primary factors: being overwhelmed by the intensity of the aggression and the extent of the damage, and not giving the healing process the required support. For example, if we make an intense physical effort, like running a road marathon, and we don't have enough training, we will likely develop knee and other joint injuries of different degrees. If we hydrate and stretch well before and after the race and take an ice bath after, the damage will be less, and the healing will be quicker and more complete.

Improving health has two main parts. First, it involves identifying, lessening, or eliminating the causes. Second, it involves increasing resilience and healing capacity by boosting demand through healthy, stimulating measures and making repair resources available.

For example, we identify and stop the cause: eating high-carb processed foods that are highly inflammatory. Then we increase our resilience by improving our digestion by fasting, chewing food well, and eating foods rich in nutrients, prebiotics, and probiotics—such as fermented foods.

In general, our resilience and healing capacity are greatly improved when we go into survival modes triggered by the habits discussed previously, particularly cold exposure, fasting, and intense exercise. If survival mode is persistent, even the genetic expression of bad genes can be suppressed or modified.

Most chronic conditions result from an unhealthy lifestyle and lack of quality essential nutrients and minerals.

It's alarming to observe that much of the adult population in Western civilization is now affected by a plethora of chronic diseases like obesity, hypertension, and diabetes. We have gained access to numerous healthy options. Yet, we still seem to be worsening, primarily due to three factors: a mismatch between lifestyle and design, exposure to novel chemicals and toxins, and abuse.

Firstly, our modern lifestyle is at odds with our biology. This is due to the progress in technology, which has presented us with novel, unnatural ways of living, as described in the previous chapters. We often opt for what is more convenient and cozier than what is best for our health. We prefer to park near the entrance of grocery stores. Or we choose to drive rather than biking or walking to a local restaurant.

Next, there are many more pollutants, toxins, and unhealthy chemicals that we are exposed to in our environment now. Technological advancement, agriculture, and other industries have introduced these into our environment. We often opt for low-quality food ordered from a chain restaurant rather than cooking or making our higher-quality dinner at home.

Last factor but not least, we misuse what is available to us. Even when what we have is beneficial to our health, if we abuse it, it can still be damaging. The truth is that we eat too frequently, too diversely, and too much.

Acute versus chronic illnesses.

An acute illness is most likely temporary, has a short-term cause, is reversible, and often has very few long-term consequences. It usually lasts days or weeks. For example, a sudden, acute infection, a broken arm, or other injury. Modern medicine can manage these well, even if it becomes severe or life-threatening.

Chronic illnesses, however, are a completely different story. They typically last months or years. Why do they persist? Because of the continuous presence of their causing factors and the establishment of an unhealthy and unproperly balanced status quo. Often, multiple complex and complicated causes contribute to a particular situation. Identifying or removing the contributing factors can be challenging.

What about symptoms?

In many acute conditions, if not severe or life-threatening, like a regular cold, indigestion, or a muscle strain, often all we need is rest, time, and treating symptoms. The body's healing capacity can take care of the rest. And because the aggression is temporary, we will end up healing ourselves. The causes of acute illnesses are usually obvious and easier to identify and remove.

With chronic illnesses, the symptoms come later and are usually just the tip of the iceberg. Because these conditions develop slowly, the body gets used to them, often maladapting. Often, we ignore or are unable to recognize the causative aggressors such as hypertension, diabetes, or cancer. In the cancer case, it often remains undetected for quite a while, as natural immunity would not recognize and respond to it. Early detection of vascular damage to various organs caused by diabetes or hypertension is difficult. Once damage to our kidney, heart, or brain becomes clinically detectable, it is often late and irreversible.

In the initial stages of chronic disease, subtle functioning disturbances are usually present, mostly asymptomatic, and difficult to identify and detect using conventional medical tests.

As imbalances or damages accumulate, subtle symptoms start to appear, sometimes even before any clinical sign or laboratory abnormalities can be detected. Often, the symptoms only occur or become significant when a new external factor or trigger pushes the person past a certain point, which I call the *awareness or tolerance point*. Hence, merely treating the symptoms of chronic diseases does not address the buildup of damage and imbalance that has been created over time, and the sickness will continue to worsen.

For example, a commonly unrecognized condition known as SIBO (small intestinal bacterial overgrowth) leads to digestive disorders caused by excessive bacteria growth in the small intestine. This condition often goes unrecognized and produces chronic digestive symptoms such as bloating, heartburn, constipation, and even chronic inflammation in other locations, such as perennial allergies or arthritis.

The symptoms of SIBO can be subtle, except when triggered or exacerbated—for instance, when the person consumes an unhealthy meal, such as frozen pizza and beer—which can lead to new digestive symptoms and a flare-up of respiratory allergies. Here. SIBO becomes a predisposing, persisting factor, and some foods become temporary, acute triggers.

Persistent predisposing factors versus temporary triggers.

Discerning between the underlying causes and the triggers that usually produce flareups is important in understanding the disease process.

In this case, we must search for the causes of each. If the symptoms are not severe, we must allow them to reflect the situation as much as possible rather than suppressing them with medications. They are a valuable way to monitor the progression of chronic illness.

Heartburn caused by stomach reflux is a common issue. Often, people try to alleviate the symptoms by taking anti-acid medications such as Omeprazole. However, a better approach would be to identify and avoid triggers such as coffee, alcohol, or eating too quickly. Additionally, it is important to address the underlying factors, such as regularly consuming unhealthy foods, overeating, or experiencing chronic high stress. Each individual often has a unique combination of triggers and underlying factors.

Identifying the causes of chronic illnesses is often difficult or impossible due to the complexity of the human mind and body.

We also need to ensure that our body's healing capacity is stimulated and enhanced, as this may be the only way we can improve when the cause cannot be removed or identified. (An example is inflammatory bowel disease like Crohn's disease or ulcerative colitis. We often cannot cure the condition, but we *can* keep it well controlled or even asymptomatic with healthier lifestyle and diet choices.)

If an acute condition is not appropriately addressed, such as an injury, then this can also become chronic, even if the original cause is gone. That's because the injured tissue can become less functional or stiffer over time. Therefore, it becomes prone to further injuries. It's like a snowball effect.

For example, the chances of reinjury after a tendon tear are especially higher if this injury is not approached with care and attention. This often occurs when the injured person returns too soon to their regular daily routine after becoming injured rather than resting and resuming functional movement progressively with qualified therapy.

Disease prevention and early detection.

Prevention is part of the standard of care today and involves recognizing and eliminating potential sources of disease. These causes are often linked to bad habits and behaviors, so we must address that. Knowing about an individual's genetic predispositions is also helpful, but lifestyle is still the primary factor. We can keep the harmful effects of genes at bay for a long time. In conventional medicine, early detection involves particular screening tests. The number of such tests is slowly increasing, too, which is excellent.

Pushing yourself to achieve optimal health can influence genetic expressions. This usually involves leaving your comfort zone, embracing difficulties, and often feeling uncomfortable. When we do this, we send a powerful message to our genes and activate our natural survival mechanisms that strive for optimal performance and the capability to adapt and thrive.

It will make us more powerful and healthier. (For instance, exercising with weights to the point of discomfort can lead to significant muscle growth in just a few weeks.) A demanding lifestyle can positively affect the genetic influences of diseases in two ways: it can reduce or inhibit the expression of undesirable genes, and it can activate beneficial genes to help you become healthier, recover from illness or injury, and thrive in life.

The modern Western culture dominates health care.

The 21st-century Western culture, which strongly emphasizes immediate gratification and comfort, also dictates in the medical field.

Unfortunately, however, the U.S. medical system has multiple flaws that need to be corrected so that we can enjoy better-quality health care. Today, the most important resources for medical advances are driven by profit instead of necessity.

According to an article in the Economist magazine, (October 19, 2013): "Modern scientists are doing too much trusting and not enough verifying—to the detriment of the whole of science and humanity."

Most medical studies cannot be replicated. With psychiatric drug studies, for instance, eighty percent are not reproducible.

This often unreliable and profit-oriented science seems too readily accepted in today's medical community. For example, a small study in Australia a few years ago made aspirin look bad. It changed, through media hype, the opinion of medical communities worldwide about the benefit of aspirin in preventing cardiovascular disease. Forget about almost 100 years of time testing and hundreds of studies showing its benefits. Why did this happen? A simple answer is this: Aspirin is cheap. And it's competing with the new, expensive blood thinners. That, as you can imagine, is an inconvenience for some.

Patient perspectives and expectations play a crucial role in shaping the modern medical landscape. However, these perspectives are often heavily influenced and manipulated by the media, food manufacturers, and healthcare product manufacturers. It's time to take charge of our health by educating ourselves about the misleading labels we come across every day. For example, the terms "sugar-free" or "diet" drinks might sound healthy, but they are actually less healthy than regular drinks because they contain artificial sweeteners instead of sugar. Instead, opt for "unsweetened" drinks for a truly healthy option. Similarly, the term "natural" is unreliable and has been misused countless times. To ensure quality, the best option is to buy directly from a reliable source such as a local small farm. While "organic" is a more reliable term, it is still far from perfect, but currently our best option when shopping in chain grocery stores.

Remember how we discussed that our primitive drives often lead to our decisions? As a reminder, we are often led by these drives because we demand immediate gratification and quick fixes and tend to disregard long-term consequences.

The same principle applies to healthcare as well.

Studies show that antibiotics are unnecessary in over thirty percent of cases (and in reality, probably over fifty percent) but they are still over-prescribed. Why? Mainly because the patient is treated like a customer. And taking antibiotics has many downsides, especially if using stronger ones or more frequently. Many patients do not realize the negative consequences associated with taking them, like digestive issues due to disturbances in the normal intestinal flora. However, they expect certainty and quick solutions—when the right approach is accepting uncertainty and having patience.

Treating the symptoms rather than the root cause is the norm nowadays.

Dealing with uncertainties that characterize the human body and mind is frustrating. Many doctors and patients prefer to ignore them and conveniently focus on treating symptoms instead of looking for a root cause, which is often uncertain in the beginning. The causes of chronic diseases are mostly ignored or marginalized.

This often fits the patient well, as dealing with the root of the problems requires more time and work, and the consequences of ignoring them are usually not immediate. Patients often want a quick fix. Taking painkillers, muscle relaxants, and sleeping pills instead of engaging in physical therapy and changing habits takes little effort and leads to immediate relief. Choosing immediate gratification versus delayed gratification is again the issue here.

These immediate remedies do not address the underlying problem; instead, they cover the root cause without ever addressing it. As you can imagine, these problems will eventually reappear once the medicines are stopped. In the initial stages, it is acceptable to use medications, provided that the primary focus remains on addressing the underlying cause. The goal should be to discontinue or reduce the reliance on medication as early as possible.

The eternal paradox is amplified in the new medical system. There's been always a conflict of interest. If all patients were to become healthy, there would be no work for the doctors.

In most instances, doctors receive better compensation for their sicker patients, so the doctor's financial interests are often not in the patient's best interest. Ideally, the less often a patient visits a doctor, the more compensation the doctor would receive.

Even worse—in recent years, with the expansion of government influence and control in medicine (such as programs like Medicare), a financial cap is imposed on each patient annually or even monthly. The amount varies depending on the overall severity of the patient's condition. The sicker the patient, the higher the yearly capped dollar amount. The capped amount is a gross approximation, which is often not realistic. If the patient requires more medical expenses and interventions than initially calculated, the remaining amount within the cap for the doctor's pay decreases. So again, we see how the doctor's financial interest conflicts with the patient's best interests.

The government is micromanaging healthcare providers to perform most efficiently in terms of quantity rather than quality. As we all know, quantity and quality often go in opposite directions. Even if their intention is to also improve quality, introducing so many regulations and more bureaucracy actually facilitates abuse and fails to resolve the healthcare crisis in the United States.

Uncertainty is more common than certainty when it comes to the human body.

We should be accepting of uncertainties, particularly in conditions that are not life-threatening, especially in primary care settings.

To illustrate this, here is a very common example of a patient coming in with acute cold symptoms. From the provider's perspective, diagnosing a virus versus a bacterium is far from 100 percent accurate, especially early on. Statistics reveal that antibiotics are overly prescribed, as between seventy and ninety percent of all upper respiratory infections are viral.

The human body is complex. Colds and infections have several variables that should be taken into consideration.

A medical provider can use the following algorithm to diagnose and treat a cold correctly. First, upper respiratory tract infections, whether bacterial or viral, manifest in many similar ways—both commonly cause mucus, fever, sore throat, headache, and cough. The color and amount of mucus are not specific to bacteria or viruses, both of which can produce swollen glands. So, how can we distinguish between the two?

We must consider how the infection spreads. In most cases, bacterial infections start and stay localized, often on one side: one ear, one eye, and one sinus. Viruses, in most cases, progress in widespread fashion over hours and days from sinuses to throat to chest, from left to right, and so on.

Second, the timing of bacterial and viral infections differs.

Viral symptoms often peak between days two and four. Symptoms usually begin to improve within three to five days and resolve entirely within seven to ten days of their initial onset.

Bacterial infections, on the other hand, may not follow a distinct peak and commonly worsen after a few days instead of subsiding.

This algorithm works well in theory. However, diagnosis is not always straightforward, as there are many exceptions due to the complexity of nature and the human body.

For example, subject to exceptions to the above rule to aid in correct diagnosis, it is not uncommon for viruses to be complicated by bacterial infections originating from our own respiratory flora. Now, the initial viral illness is transformed or complicated into a bacterial infection. This translates into a worsening or continuing the symptoms after the peak severity and extends through days seven to ten without significant improvement. For this reason, time aids in making an accurate diagnosis.

To further confuse and complicate diagnosis, the increased inflammation caused by infection can exacerbate the patient's relatively stable environment or food allergies, prolonging and worsening the disease course.

If the patient is immunosuppressed, bacteria can spread as quickly as a virus.

So, there is usually no black and white but rather many hues of gray or a mix of features. One day—hopefully soon—we will have an affordable, precise, and sensitive test that will accurately differentiate between bacterial and viral infections.

Acute urinary infections, in contrast to respiratory infections, are usually less complex. Most of them are caused by bacteria that can easily be cultured. Viruses rarely cause them. A urine culture is usually not necessary, and a blind treatment that uses a common antibiotic is often the cure. The same cannot be said concerning chronic urinary infections. Those are way more complex and come with many more variables and uncertainties.

In other medical fields—cardiology, for example—the diagnosis is often more precise. One reason is that cardiology has more advanced knowledge and technology. Diagnosing the root causes of gastrointestinal illnesses, on the other hand, is even more complex.

Getting actively involved in your health problems is crucial for successful treatment.

In my practice, I involve patients in their care to ensure understanding, accountability, and responsibility. For example, if a patient has blood pressure issues, I ask them to purchase an accurate home blood pressure monitor that has been verified against manual devices in my clinic. This is because blood pressure measurements taken during a doctor's visit are not always relevant for two reasons: first, "the white coat syndrome" (anxiety associated with being in the doctor's office).

And second, the patient needs multiple readings taken through-out the month to make an accurate observation and decision.

Blood pressure can be reactive. If the patient is stressed, anxious, tired, or slept poorly—or even if they take different over-the-counter medication—their blood pressure may temporarily increase.

Patient involvement is even more critical when diagnosing chronic digestive conditions such as heartburn, chronic bloating, diarrhea, and constipation. I minimize my patients' medication use, instruct them to make lifestyle changes, and advise them to keep food diaries. That way, they can recognize and identify triggers. Taking antacid pills daily can blind patients to possible causes and prevent them from learning from their mistakes, especially in the early stages when the situation is unclear.

The pill will often only mask the symptoms and not address the cause.

We should consider symptoms such as pain, heartburn, or spasms to be our friends. Not because they are pleasant, of course, but because they have been intelligently designed by nature to inform and protect us. They reveal *when* and *how* we tend to make mistakes. We must learn to listen to our body first, then analyze and then act and change. We need to become good detectives. If the cause is identified and cannot be changed, or if the cause is not found, then long-term medica-tion may be required as a lesser alternative.

> *"A wise man should consider that health is the greatest of human blessings and learn how by his own thought to derive benefit from his illnesses."*
>
> —Hippocrates

We are still far from understanding the causes and mechanisms of many medical conditions—despite our modern-day knowledge.

Joe, a patient in his mid-forties, has been experiencing generalized aches and pains in his small and large joints for the past two years. Despite seeing multiple specialists, including rheumatologists, and undergoing extensive workups for inflammatory autoimmune diseases such as rheumatoid arthritis and lupus, no apparent cause has been found. What's particularly strange is that Joe began experiencing these symptoms just twelve hours after having a root canal two years ago. Then, he also developed a widespread upper body rash and progressively worsening aches and pains. At first, he thought it might be an allergic reaction to medication he received during the root canal procedure, and his condition didn't respond to changes in his diet, such as eliminating inflammatory foods. Prior to the root canal, Joe was in good shape and had no complaints or medical problems. This is not an unusual case, a type of situation that I encounter almost every month.

But there are also a lot more common situations. For example, acute and chronic back pain are both common complaints and cause many people to schedule frequent doctor appointments. The abuse of painkillers for these injuries and others has become a significant cause of disability.

Here's a common scenario: A patient wakes up one morning after having an average day the day before. While reaching for an object, this person is suddenly struck by intense back pain and becomes temporarily disabled. Sometimes the cause is completely unknown, and other times it can be traced back to distant injuries from many years prior.

We try to blame the pain on a perfect storm situation—like when dehydration is compounded by inflammation-inducing foods. Or even a lack of electrolytes in the diet. When combined with a mechanical factor such as incorrect posture or movement as predisposing factors, it is not unusual for it to precipitate a crisis like this.

The mystery continues, however, as recovery may vary— there could be a quick and positive response to rest, physical therapy, and symptomatic medications, or the patient could have worsened pain and the need for aggressive treatment, including epidural shots and surgery.

The MRI (magnetic resonance imaging) results may also be surprising. There is often little correlation between the image findings and the severity of the symptoms. There are many cases in which a patient with zero history of significant back injuries is found with severe degenerative disc disease, likely due to unnatural, incorrect, prolonged sitting position, possibly compounded with a genetic predisposition, as an underlying cause. That takes many months and years to develop. And the patient may never even experience symptoms until the acute back crisis strikes.

The response of back pain to physical therapy and surgery is highly unpredictable. What can I say? Back pain is often a mystery that goes unsolved.

Another very common condition remains a mystery. One in seven women after age fifty, and many younger women, struggle with thyroid problems. These women must take thyroid medications as treatment. No one knows why thyroid issues are so common. It is commonly considered an autoimmune condition, as autoantibodies can often be detected against the thyroid gland, but there is no apparent trigger or cause. It is almost as common in men.

Each patient should be seen as a unique, complex individual rather than a standard medical case.

One of the pitfalls of modern medicine is that the physician and patient consider it pure science. In reality, an essential aspect of practicing medicine is art. The art of healing. This art needs to be practiced by both the patient and the physician.

Science will often box everything into ranges: normal ranges and abnormal ranges. But, again, there is often no black-and-white regarding our health. By default, the human body and our human nature have a lot of grays.

We can easily improve efficiency and prevent many side effects from taking medication and other substances by applying genetic testing.

Each of us has a unique, genetically designed way to handle each substance we introduce into our body.

Our body's reactions to many medications, like antidepressants, cancer treatments, and sleeping pills, are unpredictable. Most prescribed drugs are a hit or miss with respect to efficacity and side effects. Modern science is trying to solve the problem by developing genetic tests called *pharmacogenomics*. This would determine, with acceptable accuracy, how each person's body processes or metabolizes a particular drug, thus avoiding drug toxicity and futile multiple medication trials.

These genetic tests should be conducted for every individual at birth. This should be extended to common medications and the most common chemicals found in food. This approach would provide valuable insights into how each person metabolizes and responds to substances such as caffeine, alcohol, cannabis, etc.

These tests, however, are limited to the drug's metabolic pathways. For medication testing to achieve high accuracy, a test should analyze its entire path in our system. It should analyze its absorption in the digestive tract, our metabolic processes, how the drug is transported in the blood, and how we extract it through receptors at the target organs.

The way the target organs process the drug also needs to be analyzed. We are far from reaching genetic testing at this level, but knowing the metabolic pathways is helpful.

A word on genetic deficiencies, genetic tests, and the benefits of fermented foods.

Fermented foods have been used for centuries to treat various health conditions, and they have more benefits than we initially thought. Consuming fermented foods provides our body with essential vitamins and nutrients more efficiently. Here are some examples of fermented foods: kefir, plain yogurt, dry curd cottage cheese, farmer's cheese, or fermented cottage cheese, certain aged cheeses (check the label for live and active cultures), fermented vegetables, tempeh, miso, pickles, sauerkraut, kimchi, kombucha, other probiotic drinks such as beet kvass or apple cider, and other various cultured products.

Fermented foods contain high, unique nutritional values and are an excellent source of healthy bacteria. Consuming these foods is healthier than taking probiotic supplements alone. The bacteria in fermented foods break down the nutrients over time into active forms of nutrients. Sometimes, our body is incapable of doing this on its own. The bacteria do this to feed themselves; in the process, they help us to break down the same nutrients.

Methyl folates versus folic acid and other folates.

Folate is an important nutrient that is necessary for many basic cellular functions. It is found in various foods, such as vegetables, nuts, eggs, fish, and more. However, most folates found in these foods are in inactive forms, which need to be converted into the active form, 5 L-methyl folate, before they can be used by our body. This conversion process takes place in our cells and requires an enzyme that is deficient in almost eighty percent of the population.

That means that close to eighty percent of the population is unable to fully use the folates found in most foods. Most people are either partially deficient (over seventy percent) or entirely deficient (almost ten percent) in an enzyme that converts different folates into methyl L folate, the active form. This genetic deficiency is known as MTHFR (methylenetetra-hydrofolate reductase) deficiency. The official figures are less than half of the percentages I found in my clinical practice.

The defects caused by this condition have a wide range of clinical presentations. It affects various systems in our body, particularly the brain, the immune system, and the detox system. This is a significant concern, especially for the healthy development of a fetus in a pregnant woman. Insomnia, ADHD, anxiety, depression, and chronic inflammatory conditions like rheumatoid arthritis are some of the health issues caused by this deficiency. It can also lead to infertility, particularly in women, and an increased risk of blood clots in some cases. Our body's need for methyl folate increases significantly during stressful situations such as diseases and physical or mental stress. People with partial deficiency or one gene deficiency—called heterozygotes—can compensate well in average stresses present in day-to-day life. However, this is not usually the case with homozygotes, or those with double gene deficiency, as they have a severe deficiency.

In my practice, I have observed improvements in the clinical symptoms described above by using 5-methyl folate. Even mild or partially compensated deficiencies, like in heterozygotes, have shown remarkable enhancements in mood, sleep quality, energy levels, and overall sense of well-being within weeks of initiating treatment. However, the most pronounced improvements were seen in cases with severe deficiency. Furthermore, I have noticed increased resistance to common illnesses and improved inflammation, even in patients with autoimmune conditions. Many other healthcare professionals have reported similar results. Although most individuals with deficiency experience these positive effects, not everyone responds to the treatment, and the reasons for this are unknown. Supplementation with minerals and other essential nutrients may increase the response rate. However, there is still much to study and learn about folate metabolism and the essential methylation processes.

The medical community is aware of the high demand for folate during pregnancy for the mother and the baby. Therefore, folic acid has been prescribed as part of the standard of care for all pregnant women in the United States. However, we should give all pregnant women the active form, 5-L methyl folate, instead of folic acid, which is inactive and synthetic. A significant percentage of the population is not able to use folic acid completely, as stated above, and this could lead to significant negative consequences for the babies. Adding folic acid, the synthetic form, instead of the active form, 5-L methyl folate, to diverse foods, as has become common practice lately, is detrimental for those with double gene deficiency as they cannot process it at all. It should be avoided even in the majority who have only a single gene deficiency.

Milk versus other dairies.

Another example of fermented foods is yogurt or kefir, which naturally become lactose-free as the bacteria in them use up the lactose through fermentation. After age one, most individuals, except for some populations in northern Europe, experience a natural decline in lactase production as the lactase gene is switched off. This change coincides with the natural cessation of breastfeeding, as the need for lactase, the enzyme responsible for breaking down lactose in milk, decreases.

Consequently, most of us cannot break down the lactose, so drinking milk can create digestive issues, as lactose can increase inflammation in the gut. But drinking kefir or yogurt would not do the same. The bacteria in those break it down for us since they feed from lactose.

Here's the question: Thirty years from now, how many more genetic defects will we discover that result in nutrient deficiencies we most likely already have? Whatever we discover can likely be fixed today by the fermenting and nutrient-processing bacteria in fermented foods. The vast diversity and abundance of bacteria in fermented foods suggest that collectively, they are unlikely to possess significant genetic deficiencies. We would greatly benefit from studies that determine which fermented foods have what active nutrients and in what variety and amount.

Genetic testing for cancer.

Genetic tests have also shown promise in assessing the response of tumor cells to various therapeutic agents, similar to how we assess bacteria in a urine or wound culture for antibiotic resistance. These therapeutic agents, in addition to chemo and immunotherapy agents, should include natural agents such as vitamin C, cryotherapy, hyperthermia, turmeric, and salvestrol, as well as the off-label use of drugs such as hydroxychloroquine, ivermectin, fenbendazole, and so on.

However, in the United States especially, but also in other Western countries, conventional medicine has shown little interest and has been very slow to accept these precious resources.

Ignorance seemed to lie in all plans, not only toward orien-
tal medicine, unless there was a solid financial motive. The
recognition and use of these resources, especially in the United
States, will compete with current therapies and financially
threaten many large and powerful pharmaceutical companies.

**Striking the balance between quality and quantity,
safety and convenience, is necessary but challenging.**

Without creating genetically modified crops to increase
food production, many people in developing countries would
not survive. However, the food produced from these genetically modified crops tends to be less healthy and often harmful to
our health. A notable example is extensively modified wheat.
Since this is so modified, lately more than necessary, regular
consumption can lead to varying health issues. In general, the
greater the degree of genetic modification in crops, the more
profitable they become—but this profitability, which has been
excessively exploited in the past decades, often comes at the
expense of potential health problems.

Furthermore, the extensive use of pesticides and herbicides,
along with increased food processing, leads to greater profits—
but this is done at the cost of reduced nutritional value and
increased harm. The primary driver of the food industry is
financial gain, which explains its inclination to prioritize
quantity over quality, even if it undermines our health.

Similar issues, although less apparent, can also arise in the
technology field.

Developing numerous new chemicals and materials has
undoubtedly proven beneficial and, in many cases, necessary for
survival. However, it's concerning to note that there is often a
lack of rigorous safety checks and evaluations of their potential
negative impact on our health. A notable example highlighting
this issue is the widespread use of polybrominated diphenyl

ethers (PBDEs), a type of fire retardant that was extensively employed in the manufacturing of mattresses, furniture, electronics, and textiles in the United States and various other countries until the mid-2000s.

PBDEs are endocrine disruptors, meaning they can interfere with the body's endocrine system. The endocrine system regulates hormones responsible for many biological processes, including reproduction. Numerous studies have shown that exposure to PBDEs can negatively impact fertility.

Studies found that women who have high levels of PBDEs in their blood took significantly longer to become pregnant compared to women with lower levels. Other studies suggest that PBDEs can disrupt menstrual cycles and reduce sperm quality in males.

Yet, for a significant portion of our lives, we are intimately exposed to such chemicals, including eight hours a day for mattresses. This raises an important question: How strong is the correlation and causation between our regular contact with these substances and today's rise of chronic diseases of unknown cause, such as hypothyroidism, Alzheimer's, and some cancers?

Living in alignment with our biological design, free from the need for constant adaptation to new environmental changes, would be ideal. We are already born adapted to our ancestors' way of life. This way of life has changed too much over the past couple of centuries. Yes, it can be argued that we're naturally designed to adapt to modern changes—but such adaptation isn't without its burdens, challenges, and potential harm. While diversification is a natural and positive aspect of life that necessitates adaptation, there is a notable distinction between diversification driven by nature's wisdom and that driven by human intervention. The rapid advancements and vast scale of changes introduced by modern technology far surpass any natural changes we would typically encounter.

This isn't to say we should halt innovation. Rather, we should focus more on quality over quantity when introducing large-scale technologies.

From this perspective, the generations born in the past century are generations of sacrifice, as we have been extensively exposed to numerous new and often unknown harmful elements, whether these are chemical, physical, or psychological. This can provide at least a partial explanation for the rising frequency and prevalence of numerous chronic diseases at levels never seen before. However, as of 2024, technology has advanced remarkably, offering us the potential to reverse many of the detrimental changes caused by the food and technology industries in the previous decades.

The test of time and value of the old, traditional medical practices.

There are invaluable concepts that wise people have tested and added to our lifestyle over hundreds and thousands of years. These include yoga, chi-gong, tai chi, and meditation. The safety and benefits of these practices have been proven as they have withstood the test of time.

For thousands of years, one of the oldest civilizations has developed and preserved a wellness lifestyle: the traditional Chinese healing system. This advanced method of preventing and treating different chronic diseases through food combinations and daily physical practices has been practiced for thousands of years. Unfortunately, Western medicine still does not acknowledge these methods today.

Why are certain foods healthier for us to be consumed at specific hours or when combined with other specific types of food? Why does Eastern medicine consider certain aspects of health that our modern science ignores? For example, the quality of the pulse, the deposit on the tongue, the different physical and chemical properties of stools and urine, the temperature of the hands and feet, and so on.

Contemporary medicine overlooks the ancient medical knowledge of Eastern civilizations, notably China and India. Additionally, numerous traditional remedies from Europe are also sidelined.

Merging Eastern and Western medical practices would be highly beneficial. This raises the question: Is Western medicine primarily motivated by profit?

While some clinicians and select integrative or alternative centers practice a blend of Eastern and Western medicine, there isn't a comprehensive, consistently successful alternative medicine network that's widely accepted and accessible.

Though there's a large market for supplements, it's often unregulated and profit oriented. Finding a reputable brand and obtaining consistent, dependable results from supplements, especially those purchased online, is difficult. Moreover, most supplements, similar to many long-term medications, don't address the underlying causes of chronic diseases, even if they might be closer to addressing the core issue.

In our modern culture, the end of life can bring ignored, much unnecessary suffering.

There is another aspect of life—a disturbing and traumatic aspect—that modern medicine and the new culture tend to ignore. Yet almost everyone will have no choice but to face it sooner or later. That is this: how we leave this world.

Modern culture and technology have changed the way we die, but unfortunately, not in a positive way. And, of course, human nature is again to blame. Today, technology has allowed us to intervene in natural death, either by speeding it up, called euthanasia, or unnecessarily delaying it, the opposite of euthanasia. I believe they're both completely wrong, but here

I'm going to discuss the latter, as it is so common, likely to happen to most people and is completely disregarded.

I chose to write this book to help minimize suffering, especially unnecessary suffering. We cannot ignore the fact that much unnecessary suffering has occurred in the last few days or weeks of life.

Hospital doctors are not trained to communicate with or understand dying people—especially if they remain incoherent or unconscious. Most of us will likely fall into this state in the process of dying. Here's the issue: Modern technology prolongs this state far beyond its natural duration—which usually would last hours to days at most. This is artificially and needlessly postponed for days, weeks, even months, and years. The people surrounding the dying person are seeking their own comfort rather than that person's peace and comfort. This is done in hospital wards, especially intensive care units, with the help of modern life support systems, including ventilators, feeding tubes, life support medications, and other advanced technology.

Dying is a very uncomfortable experience for most people. Therefore, any artificial extensions, even if only for a few minutes, should only be undertaken if the methods are fully justified and can provide comfort. Fortunately, we do have the means to help people pass away peacefully, with minimal pain and discomfort. However, in reality, the opposite often happens. Especially after verbal communication with the dying person has ceased, assessments of their well-being are primarily based on their facial and body language, respiration, and heart rate. Unfortunately, these signs and signals of distress are often significantly altered and can no longer be trusted. This is mainly due to the effects of multiple medications and an unusually complex and prolonged clinical state that occurs in the hospital environment. Another complicating factor is the unique behavior of each individual. Pain is not the only cause of discomfort. There are other causes that we often fail to recognize or treat. For example, lack of sleep, thirst, shortness of breath, anxiety, tension, and feeling hot or cold, and so on. When ignored, these symptoms can persist and become unbearable for the dying person.

All of this can manifest differently and subtly in people who are unconscious and under the influence of multiple drugs and treatments, suffering from complex medical conditions. The longer we prolong these states, the more complicated and difficult it will be to provide treatment and comfort.

Even among medical professionals, there is a widespread misconception that being unconscious or in a coma equates to an absence of discomfort and pain. This belief, however, is fundamentally incorrect and often conveniently adopted for the sake of their own comfort.

How much can an unconscious or sedated person feel and think? How exactly do you titrate pain and anxiety medications?

Consider this: Studies show that, on many occasions, doctors tend to *undertreat* acute pain and overtreat chronic pain. Why? A bias has been produced in our country because of the abuse of narcotics in treating chronic pain. This realization explains why fear has developed regarding the overuse of comforting medications, such as narcotics and benzodiazepines, in acute care settings.

Furthermore, there is a fear that overtreatment of acute pain and anxiety may hasten or even cause death in patients. This fear is rarely justified.

We have the technology and the means but not the will to improve the dying process.

So how can we fix this? Several steps can be taken.

First, we must be aware of this situation and learn more about it.

Second, let's develop and introduce a "comfort level helmet." This "helmet" would read EEG and other brain signals and translate them into a comfort-discomfort chart. From there, we could identify the degree of stress and suffering in an individual. As technology advances and more research is conducted, we can expand our understanding of various sources and types of discomfort and their specific locations within the brain.

In a modified version, I call this helmet a *surgical helmet*. This could be used for individuals undergoing general anesthesia. The helmet would detect the brain's electric response to sedatives and other medications while monitoring vital signs such as blood perfusion, oxygen levels, pH changes, etc.

There are a few primitive technologies based on EEG signals, such as the Bispectral-Index (BIS), that monitors the level of sedation in unconscious patients. However, their utilization has been limited. Hospitals often do not make them available, nor do they actively encourage their use. Hospital policies should mandate the availability and use of such technologies.

Under-sedation is easy to assess as patients display signs of discomfort and corresponding behaviors. However, oversedation is only assessed by vital signs. Unfortunately, vital signs alone can be inaccurate and unreliable indicators of oversedation, especially in atypical settings like operating rooms.

The consequences of oversedation can be severe, fortunately mostly temporary, but sometimes permanent. Even general anesthesia for minor surgeries, such as knee or hernia surgery, can result in brain damage. This damage can manifest as memory loss, chronic fatigue, mental sluggishness, and abrupt changes that both the patient and family members easily recognize.

Other factors can damage the brain during surgery, too. Most notably, drops in blood pressure and oxygen levels. However, the precise impact of these factors on the brain could be more accurately detected in real-time using the advanced surgical helmet discussed earlier. This would allow anesthesiologists to intervene quickly and efficiently to prevent neuron loss. More research would be required for us to develop and perfect these helmets before use.

Sooner or later, each of us will benefit from creating and developing these helmets. And the necessary technology already exists. For years, we have witnessed the provision of technology that enables video gamers to connect with their computers and play games without physically interacting with buttons—simply by wearing a smart helmet. I am convinced that intelligence agencies have also developed "mind-reading" devices. They could lend some of their technology without jeopardizing their operations.

In the United States, nearly half of our medical expenses are spent in the last few weeks of our life. Sadly, a significant portion of that is unnecessary. How much money could we save simply by implementing a system that improves the dying process in all these aspects? We could make substantial strides in optimizing end-of-life care while reducing unnecessary medical costs through education programs targeting doctors, relatives, and patients.

It's not just the doctors who desire to prolong a dying person's life. The family members often share this desire as well. Due to understandable yet self-centered reasons, these relatives aspire to extend the lives of their loved ones, clinging to hopes of recovery or being in complete denial. Unfortunately, this approach only prolongs the dying process instead of extending the individual's life.

Better education is needed on the concept of non-resuscitation and comfort measures. This is especially crucial in countries like my native country, Romania, where the issue of DNR (do not resuscitate) is poorly understood and rarely addressed. As a result, many individuals nearing the end of life undergo unnecessary, prolonged, and painful resuscitation.

In summary:

Most illnesses are caused by a combination of genetic predisposition and external factors. The external factors can be attributed to an unhealthy lifestyle, exposure to new chemicals and toxins, or accidental injury. When it comes to chronic illnesses, treatment should focus on identifying and eliminating the root cause while also supporting and bolstering the body's healing ability. Most chronic illnesses have two types of causes: the *underlying cause*, which is often difficult to detect and develops slowly, often without symptoms, and the *triggers*, which tend to be symptomatic and can push us over the edge. It is essential to identify and treat both.

The new cultural bubble has also been intoxicating modern conventional medicine. The result is an explosion of chronic diseases that the medical community is unable to control or slow down, forget about curing or eradicating them. Instead of addressing the causes, it thrives financially by treating the symptoms with new medications. But you don't have to conform to this modern trend. You can break out of this toxic environment and address the causes of most chronic health issues, as described in this chapter, with a much higher chance of success.

In the next chapter, I will explain why it is so easy to destroy and so hard to create, why it is so easy to get injured or sick, and why it is so hard to recover. I will show you how everything has a purpose, even if we don't always see or understand it. Then, you will know how to apply this view to improve your health and well-being.

Chapter 14

Life and Entropy, the Battle Against Chaos

We must scale back to find our higher, constructive, or greater purpose. What is the bigger picture of our life? Why were we born in the first place?

Everything on earth is part of a system.

A leaf is part of a tree, and a tree is part of a forest.

A forest is part of the plant system, and the plant system is part of an ecosystem.

I could go on and on…

Everything that exists is also in a continuous state of *change*. Nothing stays the same. And while we do not often perceive systems in this manner, the truth is that all systems and their components are continuously moving and transforming.

This includes us as well.

The incessant battle of unseen forces.

Every system in life can change toward destruction and disintegration—or it can change toward construction and growth. At any given time, a forest may be expanding or shrinking. Some changes may not be immediately apparent to an observer. But if the images of a forest were captured over several years and played back at an accelerated speed (say, one minute), you could easily see the forest's evolution. This doesn't include the natural seasonal changes.

We can better understand the direction of change by understanding the concept of *entropy*. This is defined as:

> The measure of a system's thermal energy per unit temperature that is unavailable for doing useful work. Because work is obtained from ordered molecular motion, the amount of entropy is also a measure of the molecular disorder, or randomness, of a system.

It is the measure of a system's *chaos* or randomness. The beauty of it is that it can be applied to any kind of system, whether it is the nervous system, the planet system, or the political system. And that chaos is an indirect measurement of its capacity to work toward the system's purpose—"useful work."

Higher entropy means more chaos and changes toward disorganization or deterioration, as seen in a decaying forest. *Lower* entropy means increased order, complexity, or evolution, which is evident in a thriving forest.

Cancer is an example of this high entropy. With cancer, the cells of a malignant tumor are destructive and spread randomly. They are *chaotic*.

By comparison, a fetus, as it develops into a baby, is the opposite of a malignant tumor. A fetus is a good illustration of a highly organized, constructive system, the *opposite* of chaos.

So, what does entropy have to do with life and habits? And what does it have to do with complete health and life purpose?

The short answer is *a lot*. In the universe, widespread permanent forces constantly push us toward chaos or high entropy.

But there is a distinction between the effort required for destruction and that required for creation.

Think about the last time you injured yourself in some way. Maybe you were walking down the stairs when suddenly you slipped, twisted and sprained a knee. How easily and quickly did you get injured? Now, think about the time it took to heal—at least a month or two.

How easy is it for us to destroy and create chaos? An accidental injury leads to a state of higher entropy caused by destructive forces. These permanent, omnipresent forces push us toward injury, disease, and death. They can also lead to other forms of chaos, such as violence, crime, and war.

Unfortunately, by innately following the uneducated human mind, we are wired to bring disorder and chaos into our lives. We must be rewired and learn how to fight destructive forces by embracing and applying ancient wisdom and sound science to our daily lives.

Coping with chaos.

Over time, we created complex systems to prevent high entropy states and repair damages. Examples include the U.S. Constitution, traffic rules, state and federal laws, medicine, and so on. These systems are in place to bring and maintain order and to reduce our propensity toward damage and chaos.

Yet despite all our traffic safety measures and rules and regulations, there are an average of 40,000 deaths and millions of people disabled from car accidents each year in the U.S. alone.

Thankfully, these destructive forces do not have the upper hand. Life continues to expand, thrive, and diversify here on Earth.

So, there are powerful constructive forces that push life in the opposite direction—away from chaos and toward stability and complexity.

As we fight against chaos, it is here that we begin to discover our life's purpose.

An impossible contrast.

Have you ever considered the miracle of life? It's no wonder humans have contemplated their life's purpose across the span of centuries. Our mere existence is a miracle! And yet we remain small and frail in this infinite universe. There is little order in this immensity. Our planet stands in sharp contrast to everything we can perceive around Earth.

Life is very unusual and different. There is no resemblance or connection between life on Earth and the rest of the space we perceive with all the means of science and technology. There is no resemblance or connection between the Earth and the other known planets or stars.

Yes, life is indeed a miracle. It stands against all odds—against chaos and destruction. It has an extremely high degree of order and uniqueness.

Earth and the life it sustains have a much higher degree of diversity and complexity than the universe around us.

There must be a powerful force that created us and stands against chaos and randomness.

It is so easy to destroy and so demanding to build, yet life continues to expand and thrive.

That is why it is a miracle that life exists against all odds.

Allow me to paint a picture for you to help illustrate this.

Imagine that we stand amid a stormy ocean—but the water we are in is smooth and still, like a lake. The water is calm and pristine. And it will stay calm, despite the powerful storms, currents, and winds. And the calm water is very different in color, temperature, and clarity.

What is the chance that this calm water would randomly appear and last? How big is the force that could allow this to occur and persist?

This also reminds me of a quote from the astronaut James Irwin:

"The Earth reminded us of a Christmas tree ornament hanging in the blackness of space. As we got farther and farther away, it diminished in size. Finally, it shrank to the size of a marble, the most beautiful marble you can imagine. That beautiful, warm, living object looked so fragile, so delicate, that if you touched it with a finger, it would crumble and fall apart. Seeing this has to change a man, has to make a man appreciate the creation of God and the love of God."

There must be a powerful intent to organize, create, evolve, and multiply in such a unique and organized fashion. Still, we have one essential important feature in common with the rest of the universe. It is the propensity for diversity, movement, and change. We are also permanently at risk of becoming part of randomness and chaos and destruction, of becoming dust.

And inevitably, at least a part of us does return to dust.

Our purpose is the reason we are here.

To understand our life's purpose, we must take a moment to refresh the definition of a *system*:

"A regularly interacting or interdependent group of items forming a unified whole, such as a group of … objects or an organization forming a network especially for distributing something or serving a common purpose."

Voila! The purpose must come first, as the system is created *after* (in a double sense) the purpose!

So, what do I mean when I say, "*Our purpose is the reason we are here*"?

To answer this, take a moment to think about the streets, roads, and highways in a traffic network system. They work together for a common purpose, right? They were created to help us travel quickly and efficiently.

Now, think about a single microscopic cell in your body and its common parts (plasma membrane, cytoplasm, ribosomes, and DNA). They also work together for a common purpose.

Life is a system whose purpose is to become, by itself, more complex, more organized (lower entropy), able to reproduce, survive, conserve, and evolve. The human being is at the top of evolution, representing the highest complexity (lowest entropy), on this planet.

Entropy is the measure of a system's chaos or randomness. And that chaos is an indirect measurement of its capacity to work toward the system's purpose.

So, while discovering *your* purpose, I challenge you to ask yourself: *What if the purposeful use of my life is the reason my life came into being?*

If we were created for constructive purposes, why do we often move toward destruction and suffer unnecessarily?

In short, it is our immature conscious mind to blame.

Our body, internally and biologically, automatically follows the inner inherited intelligence of nature; we call it *life's mind*, which is protective and superior, as opposed to the human mind. Our body aligns subconsciously with the lower entropy of life's constructive forces.

But as conscious beings, through the human mind, we gained the ability to alter our natural balance and escape its protective effect. Once this happens, we become more exposed and vulnerable to the natural destructive entropic forces that dominate the universe.

In other words, when the human mind doesn't align with the protective, intelligent life's mind, we become vulnerable and likely will end up with unnecessary suffering.

High entropy is seen as disorder. One illustration is disease, which is a less stable state, one of increased disorder compared to a healthy state. This means that the healthier we are, the higher our body's stability, complexity, and order. Death represents a significant decrease in order—death is chaos.

The same applies to our human psyche—our mind and emotions.

Anxiety, for example, is a higher chaotic state than being calm and relaxed. Anxiety decreases our system's capacity to work toward a constructive purpose. The entropy of our psyche, our emotions, is separate from the entropy of our body. But the state of one indirectly affects the other.

Are you asking the right question?

Undoubtedly, some aspects of suffering in our lives occur beyond our control—like an accident, for instance. And, of course, there is no escaping death. It will come to all of us eventually.

But we can make constructive decisions to help us evolve and thrive rather than just survive.

You see, we were not created to simply get by day-to-day. We were created to thrive by living a healthy, full, creative, and vibrant life.

It is important to note that the more stable a system is, the more likely it is to fulfill its purpose.

Keep in mind that the degree of disorder—or entropy—is a characteristic of a system. It is not a *force*. We can only measure the *effect* these destructive or constructive forces have on a system. We cannot detect them directly.

Take gravity, for instance. We cannot detect gravity's force directly; however, we can see its effect on every object and person. We measure it through its effects.

These constructive and destructive forces affect all systems and all of life. They are not limited to physical and biological systems. This battle between entropic forces exists at multiple system levels—from the cellular level to the whole-body system, to relationships, to the environment, to the social scale, and to the global Earth scale.

These natural forces transcend all systems. This gives them the power to continually influence each of us at all levels and impact our physical bodies, minds, and emotions. They transcend from the physical, biological realm to the psyche, emotional, and spiritual realms.

So, what's the good news?

The good news is that we have the power within us to bring about positive, constructive changes.

One example is our power to choose the way we handle a dispute—resolving it with our words or using physical force.

Do you see the conflict that we constantly find ourselves in? At any given moment, various forces might push us in conflict-ing directions, some constructive, some destructive, and some neutral. The resultant force will move us in only one of these three directions.

Your stomach growls, but you know that dinner is an hour or so away. You feel hungry and irritated. So, what do you do? Do you wait for dinner? Or do you reach for cookies or potato chips?

Many have created a habit of reaching for junk food be-tween meals. This decision is often driven by stress and the need to relieve frustration. But in a short time, this habit can lead to significant weight gain and associated increased fatigue, allergies, and reduced mental clarity. In the long term, these choices can cause diabetes and vascular disease.

So perhaps that old saying is true in that we don't make our decisions. *Our decisions make us.*

The hierarchy of systems and the power of purpose.

Let's circle back to the beginning of this chapter. Remember how I said that everything in life was created with a purpose? You may see evidence of this in your body and nature. A system usually works to support the superior system to which it belongs. The primary purpose for the existence of a subsystem is to help the superior system function.

In the forest example I gave earlier, the leaves support the tree by accessing needed light and carbon dioxide. In the human body, the primary purpose of neurons is to serve the nervous system, and the main purpose of the nervous system is to support brain function. The brain's main purpose is to enable the body to function and survive.

So, everything that exists is part of a system and is moving in a direction that can be quantified and qualified from an entropic order/disorder perspective. Everything has a purpose and is a consequence of a purposeful movement or change.

We can trust that all of life was created for a reason. Every system—and all components of it—were designed to work toward fulfilling its purpose.

The purpose creates the system. The system does *not* create a purpose.

And each of us has the potential to work toward this purpose.

So, I leave you with a final question:

What decisions will you make today to fulfill this constructive purpose of your life?

In summary:

The nature of life is that everything alive is part of a system. Systems are ordered hierarchically, so each system is made of subsystems whose purpose is to serve the superior one. Nothing stays unchanged; all systems are being transformed at any given moment in two possible directions: toward organization and order or disintegration and disorder, toward its purpose or away from it. There is a universal propensity toward chaos and destruction. It is much easier to destroy or damage than to build or repair, but still, life continues to evolve and thrive as there are inner forces that make that happen. Entropy is a concept that permits us to assess the level of order or disorder of a system and its capacity to serve its purpose. It is a useful perspective that can be applied to any level of life, whether it is a cell, a body, or a society.

Chapter 15

Purpose Drives Everything

Can you recall the last time you had to remain still for several hours on a plane or in a car? How did your muscles feel afterward? Most people will claim that their muscles were stiff. This happens to me whenever I drive a long distance without stopping to stretch and move. A muscle that doesn't fully and regularly contract will stiffen and shrink fast.

If you've ever had your arm or leg immobilized for a couple of weeks following an injury, you know it causes your muscles to waste. Within a few weeks, your muscles can shrink to nearly half their usual size. The old adage "use it or lose it" fits this scenario exactly.

You may wonder—what, exactly, does this have to do with purpose?

There is a hierarchy of purposes in all systems. Consider that muscle again. A muscle's purpose is to contract, and the purpose of that is to allow us to move and lift. Why must we move and lift? When it comes to survival, the purpose of moving is to allow us to find food or run away. In this example, survival is the superior purpose; survival is the drive and the designer. The lower purposes—contracting, moving, or lifting muscles—are aligned with the superior purpose.

So—the muscles serve the limbs, the limbs serve the body, the body serves the brain, and so on.

Do you see the hierarchy of purpose here?

Purpose gives life to everything. Purposes create and drive movement and change.

We've already discussed what a purpose is: a reason, an objective, an ambition, and a plan. Next, we'll talk about the types of purposes that exist, what purpose does, and how we react to purpose. After that, you will be prepared to know where to look for meaning and how to choose it.

Purpose and human consciousness.

Have you ever stopped to appreciate the luxury we humans have of being aware of purposes? It's something that we tend to take for granted. But if you think about it, having a purpose is an incredible advantage! Our conscious mind gifts us with the capacity to create new purposes. Animals do not have this privilege. Dogs, for example, live driven by purposes, but they are unaware of them. They cannot create new purposes.

We aren't often aware of our purpose. Regardless, purpose is what drives us. We are designed and driven by it, even if we aren't aware of it. Our awareness does not affect most purposes, except the ones we create.

Purposes will continue to exist without our acknowledgment; we cannot exist without them.

For example, think about sleep—a simple, universal habit—yet one with a vital purpose. Sure, you may have gone through seasons of life where you lacked optimum sleep. But it's impossible for our body to carry on daily activities with zero sleep. In fact, without sleep, we will die in less than a week.

The purpose of sleep is to allow our bodies to recover and regenerate. It is part of our design and one that we cannot change.

All life has a purpose.

Everything that exists is part of a system, and everything that exists has a purpose. The purposes of the parts are different from that of the whole. Ultimately, though, there is one that is the mother of all purposes.

Many people call this supreme purpose God. John the Apostle writes, "In the beginning was the Word, and the Word was with God, and the Word was God" (John 1:1). According to the Greek translation (John's gospel was written in Greek), the word "Word" is *logos*, which means reason or plan.

Purpose is reason in action. A plan implies purpose and reasoning. The purpose of easier transportation and transmission gave birth to the discovery of the wheel and the axle, and their powers transformed mankind.

So, the purpose comes before creation; the purpose creates the system. This means that the universe came after its purpose. So, what was before the universe? The Creator. The Purpose.

God.

We could easily replace "Word" with "Purpose" without changing the meaning. "In the beginning was the [Purpose], and the [Purpose] was with God, and the [Purpose] was God."

The purpose of creating the human being.

Have you ever wondered why we were created in the first place?

In the Bible, we learn that God intends for humans to manifest and fulfill their creative, constructive abilities and capabilities. We were designed to do more than simply survive. God didn't bring us into existence just so that we could struggle our way through this life.

Rather, we were made in God's image. Why? So that we can thrive. Evolve. Explore. Expand. And create. When we use our Creator-given abilities to their fullest, this involves that we limit our destructive nature. We were made to be creative and productive, just like our Creator is.

When we discover and learn how nature and the universe work, we begin to learn more about the Creator and His purposes. Science aims to do all of the above, but it names the Creator "nature" or "the universe."

It's an honor to know that our Creator gave us the capacity to be aware of our creation. Why? Because that means He wants to connect with us! It also means we must share common traits and qualities with our Creator. Think about it: We would be less likely to connect and communicate if we were totally dissimilar. Right?

It's clear throughout most religions' scriptures that God's purpose for us is that we would have a relationship with Him. And just like any healthy relationship, both parties involved must be free to make choices without being controlled—which is why He gave us our conscious mind. The closer we grow to God, the more we understand Him and His creation. And the stronger our relationship is with Him, the better off we become because we will follow our higher purpose in life.

The hierarchy of purposes.

Unfortunately, human nature often pulls us in different directions. We have desires that draw us further away from our true purpose and from our relationship with God. This, of course, is often destructive and causes unnecessary suffering because we are essentially moving away from our high purpose.

We often create new purposes that are unaligned with God's purpose for us. This is the downside of having choices and free will.

Have you ever wondered what drives you to make certain decisions?

In practice, everything we do voluntarily falls into one of these three categories:

- To fulfill a basic need or purpose (like sleeping or eating).

- To fulfill a desire beyond basic needs (representing most of our efforts, like being financially successful).

- To rest, enjoy life, etc. (This category includes activities for various, mostly neutral purposes—such as observing nature, relaxing, listening to music, and so on.)

Think about the very last thing you did before opening this book. Which category did it fall under? If we took the time to examine our daily decisions, we would notice that each could be assigned to one of these categories.

Our desires are driven by purposes that can be aligned, neutral, or opposed to the higher purpose that designed us.

But we need to be careful. We often hijack basic needs and abuse them. For example, when we overeat or we overvalue sexuality, our choices become driven by manipulated, abused primitive drives. Instead, we should allow our intentions to become operated by good ideas, principles, and purposes and not only by primitive drives.

We must recognize that having a conscious mind makes us manipulative. We hijack our primitive drives and use them beyond their natural scopes, leading us far away from our needs. We begin to confuse and replace *needing* with *wanting*.

We often trick ourselves into believing that a good idea triggered the drives—expressed by feelings—when, in reality, it occurred the other way around. Through rationalization, for example, we often look for ideas that fit our primitive drives and falsely claim that the idea came before the drive.

Sometimes, it's difficult to discern which came first, the idea or the feeling. To see how this works, pretend you accidentally walked into a mobile animal shelter and are introduced to a little puppy ready for a family. This puppy grabs your heart immediately. You buy the puppy without even considering what all this responsibility entails. So, on the drive home, you tell yourself all the reasons why you can handle keeping a puppy. Your emotional drive triggered this buying decision, and then your mind tries to follow to rationalize and justify it.

Or let's say you make an untraceable but significant mistake at your job. Your heart wants to hide it, preserve your pride, and avoid a shameful situation. But your conscience and rational mind urge you to disclose it. You decide to ignore your feelings and come clean with your boss. That decision was motivated by your mind and the noble idea of telling the truth.

Missing the higher purposes.

Our human mind can be either a blessing or a curse. We decide which to embrace. Our intelligence elevates us above other animals; we are more efficient and powerful. But as creators of trivial purposes, our own created purposes often pull us away from the highest purpose—the one that designed us.

A Christian would know this well. This principle is addressed in the first and second commandments found in Exodus 20:4-5:

"You shall have no other gods before Me. You shall not make for yourself an idol, or any likeness of what is in heaven above or on the earth beneath or in the water under the earth. You shall not worship them or serve them."

Wouldn't you agree that, in our Western culture, we have an endless number of idols? These might not look like carved statues; instead, they come in the form of sports stars and Hollywood celebrities. We tend to place too much importance on superficial aspects of society, such as looks, money, power, or fame. Lust and sex become new idols we often worship subconsciously.

With the number of divorces so high in America today, consider the choice many married couples face: to break up and divorce, leave their children without two parents—or prevent a breakup by controlling primitive drives, such as lust or pride. Marriage's purpose is to make us stronger and better, not simply to have kids and avoid being alone.

If you're married or have ever been married, perhaps you'd agree that marriage is a serious but constructive challenge. It is a challenge that, if we cope with it well, will help us not only survive but also thrive. And healthy long-term relationships require compromise, patience, character, self-control, and so on.

Living by our design.

If you're on the quest to discover your purpose, I want to encourage you with this truth: Your purpose has already been designed. We were created to align our lives to higher purposes. We were designed, in a particular way, to grow, evolve, and thrive. So this means we don't have to struggle so much in this journey toward different purposes; instead, we should align with the Creator's design for us. When we chase after new, self-created ideals, we distract ourselves from what is best, and we could get hurt.

Let me give you an example. At a basic level, we were designed to sleep at night and to be active during the day. Thus, night-shift workers bear a significant increase in cardiovascular disease due to the stress of adapting to the opposite schedule.

Running on concrete for an extended period is another example of going against our design. This is a "purpose" we have created for ourselves; however, it is often an unnecessary burden to our body. Since it goes against our design, it should be avoided. Doing this kind of running consistently, as I explained in the earlier chapters, can destroy our knees. Biking for long periods, too, can affect the blood supply and result in erectile dysfunction. We've tried to cope and adapt by creating running shoes, bike seats, and heavily padded biking pants. On the other hand, running on a trail in the woods is the best and fits our design perfectly, so we would not need any special adaptation in this situation.

Now, let's think about this on a grander scale. We have also been designed to believe in a superior force, to follow that force, and to submit.

An atheist believes in the power of science. Any prosperous society follows an ideal, an idol that gives them life, purpose, and unity. Men without an ideal and robust purpose to follow tend to become lost and weak.

In summary:

As there is a hierarchy of systems, there is also a hierarchy of purposes, as systems are created to serve and support the superior system. So, on the top of the pyramid of systems, there is the highest purpose, after which the most superior system is created to serve. All systems are designed according to their purposes. Their capacity to fulfill their purpose is directly correlated with their health and stability. That also applies to humans. Cancer is an example of an unsteady destructive state of a body system as opposed to a fetus, which is an example of a stable and constructive one. This perspective can be usefully applied to any person's state, whether it is physical, mental-emotional, or spiritual. We need to make sure that what we do does not go against our design and higher purpose, against health and stability.

Chapter 16

The Ultimate Purpose

"The purpose of existence is the seeking of purpose."

—Plato

What is the ultimate purpose?

Here's a thought that may have crossed your mind:

What is the purpose of a virus?

From a scientific perspective, a virus's purpose is to exist, manifest, survive, multiply, and diversify. The question is, though, do these features make up a virus's ultimate purpose? I dare to say *no*. I believe that viruses are parts of a bigger system, a system with various purposes. In nature, we call it scientifically *ecological balance*.

We are far from understanding all purposes that drive and shape different ecological systems.

For instance, we don't yet understand gravity's purpose. We may never figure it out. You could say that gravity lacks purpose. That's possible, sure, but very unlikely. Or you may incorrectly state, from a narrow perspective, that the only purpose of gravity is to prevent all objects from falling off the earth. But we also know that the complex interaction among different planets, stars, and galaxies involves gravity.

So, what is the ultimate purpose that created all other purposes—the one that designed all superior systems? Is it survival? And if not, then how high is survival in the hierarchy of systems and purposes?

As you can see, this can become a complex subject. It gets even more difficult when we notice how some purposes can appear contradictory—but that's only because we do not understand them completely. Consider migratory birds, such as Canadian geese. They fly thousands of miles every year, and half of them die during the journey. Why is that?

Florida egrets, on the other hand, are not migratory. Their lives are much easier. With one quick movement, they can capture a fish in their beak. Often that fish is a big enough meal for the whole day. Compared to the geese, the egrets' existence seems unfair, doesn't it? You could also say it's unfair compared to that of a woodpecker, which spends hours working to eat only a few insects.

But, again, our human understanding is limited.

Efficiency versus diversification.

Is our mere purpose to survive—or is there a superior purpose that drives us all?

Recently, scientists have begun to copy biological models to create the most efficient systems. This branch of science is known as *biomimetics*. Some newer solar panel designs are derived from the use of this science. We discovered that the sunflower has a much more efficient angle and shape to capture the sun's rays than most plants. That is nature's intelligent mind. So, some of the new solar panels are now modeled to mimic the sunflower's design, and they are thirty percent more efficient than the previous flat ones.

Still, while the sunflower is perfectly designed to capture solar energy efficiently, many other flower species are not designed similarly. Thus, they are less efficient at capturing solar energy. That is also nature's intelligent mind. Is this a contradiction?

Does this variation, this inequality, in design mean, maybe, that survival is *not* the most important purpose of life?

Thousands of types of flowers, leaves, birds, and animals exist, and their efficiency with respect to survival varies substantially. Remember, a butterfly's life may last only a few days or weeks, a worker bee lives just a month or two, while sea turtles can live a hundred years and there are giant tortoises living nearly two centuries.

If survival were the ultimate purpose, even when taking into consideration the huge variety of regional conditions, one would expect a lot more similarities in design among species driven by the ideal design for survival.

So, back to the original question: Could it be that a superior purpose supersedes survival?

Diversity, perhaps?

Higher meanings.

When we renounce efficiency and embrace diversity to create, we call it art. Nature is God's art. The diversity within nature is truly impressive; it is infinite.

So, one of the higher meanings in our own life should be to create and diversify in a constructive direction. We should seek to discover our own creative gifts and strengths and then develop and use them frequently, actively, purposely, and positively. We should also work to help others do the same.

We create cars, buildings, airplanes, and ships that follow the most efficient design known (at the time) because we are mainly driven by *efficiency*. Therefore, the diversity of manmade design is very limited compared to the diversity in natural design or even art. There is a lot of repetition in manmade technological designs. Take car designs, for example. Each generation includes cars that are very similar in design, structure, and operation.

Why should we want to follow the status quo when we were created to diversify?

Let's think about the remarkable achievements that mankind has accomplished in all fields, ranging from arts and sports to technology and biology. These accomplishments only came when we embraced creativity and diversity, and someone *pushed the status quo.*

We explored. Developed. Innovated. We pushed our own limits to create something new, out of the ordinary.

No one would have believed fifty years ago that a human being could run a marathon, 26.2 miles, in under two hours. Mankind continues to break world records, our own records, year after year. And every year brings the release of millions of new songs, paintings, and books. And every year, millions of new patents are filed.

In our society today, due to our openness and interest in exploration and creativity, we have the privilege of living in good conditions and being exposed to more opportunities than ever before. This has brought about, in turn, an explosion of our creativity.

Who could argue that this—bringing creativity and constructive diversity into this world—is not a good purpose?

Multiple perspectives, same meaning.

We are meant to create the perfect conditions for human beings to reach their maximum, constructive potential. We must continue to evolve and create while limiting our *destructive* nature (which only brings suffering and chaos).

This purpose is what the Christian God and the gods of other major religions seek to achieve. Science attempts to achieve this as well. A spiritual man limits his destructive nature by following specific advice from his spiritual texts and the spiritual culture of his time. An atheist follows specific advice from scientific books and his contemporary culture. The results are similar; the purpose is the same. It is the *form and the endpoint* that differ.

Those who experience a sense of purposelessness may also encounter the subsequent depression that often accompanies it. We can become nonfunctional when lacking purpose in life. This explains why retired people are sometimes unhappy. They've lost their former routine and daily purpose.

From the perspective of entropy, humanity's purpose is to *reach the highest level of organization* (lowest entropy).

For hundreds of thousands of years, we lived as Homo sapiens without much evolutionary change. We simply existed to multiply and survive. It was only when we achieved our human mind, or consciousness, and were able to recognize our higher purpose, that we evolved quickly toward it. I believe it corresponds metaphorically to the biblical story about Adam and Eve eating from the forbidden tree—the tree of knowledge of good and evil (or the tree of consciousness and free choice). This is the moment when a true relationship between man and God started.

Therefore, the objective of life could be to determine the specific path that fulfills the highest purpose and actively pursue that direction.

Interesting concept, isn't it?

If I am created by the Maker, as opposed to randomly appearing, then I would want to know *why* I was created and what the Maker wants from me. We need to find out what our Creator wants from us—in general and for each individual in particular.

That is what we should value the most. For Christians, we can find the general purpose in the Bible. If we do, then we may find the individual meaning while working to have a more direct, closer relationship with God.

This involves spreading and applying God's wisdom in every way we can, and then translating it into our everyday lives.

From the spiritual perspective, we are made to be creative lenses for our souls.

"We are not human beings having a spiritual experience. We are spiritual beings having a human experience."
—Pierre Teilhard de Chardin, a French Jesuit priest, paleontologist, and philosopher

Our physical presence on this planet has the purpose that our souls connect and interact with God's other physical creations as well as with God Himself. It is part of the process of knowing and relating with God. It is also a way souls connect and interact. The resulting experiences enrich our souls, as souls cannot directly experience the physical realm.

The human conscious mind further enriches and diversifies the physical experience. Of course, these experiences can be destructive, too, as we have the freedom to do so. Freedom, acquired through our conscious mind, is required for the sake of expression and diversification.

The illuminated minds of mankind.

We owe what we have today—all our advances in technology, culture, science, and art—to the geniuses of our species, who together total only a few hundred people. Without them, we would probably still be in the Middle Ages or back in prehistoric times.

How did these people—such as Isaac Newton, Leonardo da Vinci, Hippocrates, and so on—achieve such accomplishments and innovations?

Because they were creative and inquisitive. They kept asking *why* and *how*. They searched for revelations, answers, and inspiration.

The speed of our Western society's evolution, due to rapid advancements in technology over the past 200 years, indicates that *we are designed to fulfill our purpose to create and diversify*. On Earth, humanity is at the top of the pyramid of evolution, complexity, and diversity. We can create the most complex, organized, and stable systems (the lowest entropy or the highest order).

Two directions, yet many ways.

As previously discussed, being healthy is a more stable and lower-entropy state than being sick. So, obviously, healthier people have higher constructive potential and are more likely to perform better.

A lower entropy system has a greater potential to perform its purpose and the work it was created to do.

We learn both from the Bible and from history that, since the very beginning, the human mind often has been destructive. Sure, we continue to evolve toward a higher purpose as a species, as a whole. But as individuals, we, unfortunately, seem very much the same.

Two main overlapping purposes drive everything in the universe. The first, more general purpose is to manifest, change, and diversify *in various directions*. This includes gravitating toward destruction and chaos. It cannot be avoided.

The second purpose is to diversify, manifest, and change *in a specific direction*, as toward higher complexity and order. This second purpose is essential for maintaining life on Earth (and likely for any other civilization). At a higher level in the purpose hierarchy, humans have a choice. Our choice is to move toward either more complexity and stability or toward chaos.

In summary:

A *system* serves a purpose, and a *purpose* designs a system. That means the same thing. The purpose comes first; it is the *designer* of the system. The existence of purpose implies the existence of both consciousness and reason. So, we can conclude that *consciousness existed before the material world.*

We are made and driven by purposes that we do not always completely understand. This is what keeps us alive and well and helps us thrive. To reach complete health, we must purposefully move toward our intrinsic higher purposes instead of creating insignificant divergent purposes. Unfortunately, our mind's nature tends to influence us to do the latter.

We are meant to create the perfect conditions for us to reach our maximum, constructive potential. We must continue to evolve and create while limiting our *destructive* nature (which only brings suffering, disease, and chaos).

From the spiritual perspective, we are made to be creative lenses for our souls so we can better connect and relate to our Creator, His creations, and our highest purpose: God.

In the final chapter, I will explore the impact of our de-structive nature on society at large, as well as present a solution that has been proven effective throughout history.

Chapter 17

We Need Good Systems to Protect Us from Ourselves

This chapter aims to analyze and demonstrate how human nature's flaws manifest at the global level, affecting every one of us. It also provides potential modern solutions inspired by ancient wisdom.

We must be clear about how our individual problems— particularly our natural tendencies to abuse—are reflected in society and interpersonal relationships. Most laws, regulations, and constitutions were initially created to keep us in check and to minimize this harm. They were written for the good of our society. Unfortunately, over time, these instruments intended to establish order have been used as tools for some to take advantage of others. But what can we expect when too much power falls into the hands of a few?

The fundamental aspects of human nature have remained largely unaltered since ancient times. Looking back at our history offers an invaluable lesson.

There is no evidence to support the notion that we, as individuals, have improved over the past millennia. In fact, the opposite is true. As humans, we persistently stumble and fall. We veer off course and inflict harm upon ourselves and others. Our choices often limit and harm us, and we witness or experience various harmful behaviors, including drug abuse, domestic violence, crime, murder, and wars. Unfortunately, these failures are ongoing and seem inevitable. Our flawed, mind-manipulated human nature and weak or easily deceived moral compasses lead us astray. We have established laws precisely—to provide stabilizing systems that protect us. And we need God to navigate these challenges effectively.

Since man walked the Earth, inflated desires have led us down unhealthy and harmful paths. In the past few decades, the new culture aided by technological progress has encouraged and enhanced our destructive side to manifest and harm. It also ignores and erases most previous generations' cultural values. We need a cultural revolution. Self-destructive behavior harms families, communities, and even nations. So, what is the solution? What can prevent this harm? The answer is *fear*, sometimes inspiration, sometimes reasoning, and sometimes love—and these *after* the proper culture is established.

The individual's propensity to move closer to God in times of crisis and away from Him in times of prosperity is reflected in society, as in the cycles of democratic society evolution described by the Scottish historian Sir Alexander Fraser Tytler in 1787. During prosperity, people not only become less spiritual, but they also tend to water down their morals. They often begin to abuse their power. Why? Because the more you have, the more you want, and a vicious circle continues. This cycle of leaving and returning to spirituality in our individual lives is rooted in our nature.

We are often reactive, shortsighted by immediate gratifications, and looking through a distorted lens. We completely lose sight of the higher purpose; we become our own gods. (All this is presented in more detail in the Human Nature chapter.)

Tytler wrote:

"A democracy cannot exist as a permanent form of government. It can only exist until the voters discover they can vote themselves largesse [generous amounts of money] from the public treasury. From that moment on, the majority always votes for the candidates promising the most benefits from the public treasury, with the result that a democracy always collapses over loose fiscal policy, which is always followed by a dictatorship. The average age of the world's greatest civilizations has been two hundred years. These nations have progressed through this sequence:

> *From Bondage to Spiritual Faith;*
> *From Spiritual Faith to Great Courage;*
> *From Courage to Liberty;*
> *From Liberty to Abundance;*
> *From Abundance to Complacency;*
> *From Complacency to Apathy;*
> *From Apathy to Dependence; and*
> *From Dependence Back into Bondage.*

Because of our human nature tendencies that we discussed in Chapter 12, we now understand why and how this evolution from one stage to another occurs naturally. As I write this in 2024, our nation in America is in the *apathy* phase, leading toward *dependence*.

Now, let's break down this progression of the rise and fall of nations.

"From Bondage to Spiritual Faith": Societies usually begin in a state of bondage. They are held captive by their ruler(s). Soon, this control prompts the people to break away and seek freedom and liberty found in adhering to spiritual faith.

"From Spiritual Faith to Great Courage": As people grow in their faith, they obtain courage and boldness found outside of themselves.

"From Courage to Liberty": The courage the people obtain prompts them to break away from bondage and step into freedom.

"From Liberty to Abundance": This newfound freedom prompts the people to work hard, and this reaps prosperity for the nation.

"From Abundance to Complacency": The generations that had been in bondage have passed. These new generations take advantage of their liberty and abundance by failing to keep up their hard work ethic. This, in return, leads to complacency.

"From Complacency to Apathy": At this point, society as a whole develops a general apathetic attitude toward their freedoms. They do not try to continue to maintain the strong character or work ethic that led to this freedom. Taking advantage of their liberty, people tend to develop a self-centered nature.

"From Apathy to Dependence": This is when society begins to lose its freedom. Because of their self-absorbed and lazy tendencies, society begins to rely on the government. And crooked politicians will undoubtedly use this to their advantage. They do this by making it so that people have no choice but to rely on the government for their needs, and these people will continue to vote for this political party because of their free gifts.

"From Dependence Back into Bondage": Freedom is officially lost at this point. Now, society is pliable in the hands of those with the greatest power. And the nation is precisely where it was at the beginning of this cycle.

This natural cycle is summarized like this: Hard times create strong men; strong men create good times; good times create weak men; and weak men create hard times.

The Founding Fathers never intended for America to become a democracy. That is evident in the Constitution. But because of our human nature, society has progressed on the above cycle; in the process, we have drifted away from being a republic.

Thanks to modern technology, politicians' level of control and resilience is dramatically higher today than in any other historical period, so the bondage/pre-revolution phase may be delayed or even prevented. We may remain in the dependence/captive phase for a very long, painful time.

As a nation, we cannot remain where we are today. We need discipline and good culture, and we especially need spirituality to rescue us from the messes we have made. Nonspiritual laws, regulations, and systems cannot save us as individuals. Sure, they might save a society from destruction, but they cannot save the *individual*. And ultimately, a society comprised of failed individuals is a failed society. Because of our self-destructive nature, we need both personal laws that are moral and spiritual, plus social laws and regulations such as those preserved in the U.S. Constitution. But we cannot allow the state to regulate the intra-individual issues—that is communism or tyranny. The state may *only* be allowed to partially regulate inter-individual social matters.

In an ideal world, if we could completely solve our personal issues—which are psychological and spiritual in nature—then we may also be able to solve our interpersonal issues. However, as you probably know, this is not possible. Therefore, interpersonal laws and regulations are needed to control the failure of intrapersonal matters. They work mainly by threats, so we fear the consequences of breaking these laws.

Think of it this way: The U.S. Constitution and its proxy can protect society from the individual but still cannot protect the individual from himself.

We are known as the "land of the free." Let's take a brief moment to evaluate what this *freedom* stands for in America. Well, what is it, exactly, that we are set free from?

Are we set free from…

- Ourselves as instinctual animals? No, that is a spiritual issue and is impossible to achieve entirely.
- Our own destructive nature? Yes, partially, but only in inter-individual relations.
- A dictator-imposed regime? Absolutely. History has demonstrated this so far.
- Terrible ideas that have led to horrible experiments like fascism or communism? Yes, but we are in danger of losing it with the creation of new waves of utopic thinking of globalism and woke culture.

Most ideas, including new ones, concerning how to fix human nature problems are likely fueled by ego, pride, greed, cultural ignorance, and a lack of historical knowledge. This is a natural, yet very dangerous, truth for men. When strong impulses are elicited, rationalization and justification follow.

Barry Schwartz, a psychologist, said: *"False ideas about human beings will not go away if people believe that they're true. Because if people believe that they're true, they create ways of living and institutions that are consistent with these very false ideas."*

As I mentioned, there is little to add to what has been discovered about human nature and society. This is why it's best to tweak and make minor adjustments rather than radical changes to these laws and regulations. History has proved that these new, "sound fair" ideas are dangerous when rooted in concepts contradictory to our fundamental nature.

Take, for example, the idea that we should all be equal. The idea proposed suggests the suppression of diversity and inequality across races, sexes, cultures, and other various values. It's suggested that they should all share the same, or at least similar, limits. In other words, "unfairness" should not even exist in any form. Within this emerging woke culture, the focus shifts not only toward ensuring equal opportunities for all individuals but also toward striving to assure equal outcomes through equity principles, and merit is less important, if at all. Do not be confused by the "pro-diversity" term of the woke ideology that this new destructive culture hijacked. As the famous Greek philosopher Aristotle said over 2,000 years ago: *"The worst form of inequality is to make unequal things equal."*

We should abide by natural laws and not dismiss them.

Hopefully, by now, you can see that nature is not fair. Diversity is a higher purpose, even beyond survival in the hierarchy of purposes. Life, like nature, is unfair to humans too. By default, our genes seem to produce the greatest injustice out there, which seems wrong, but only if viewed from a limited perspective.

Diversity supersedes fairness and even survival. Knowing that, we can then accept the truth that unfairness is natural, unavoidable, and unstoppable.

Human nature is designed to pursue self-interest. To avoid potential destruction at the societal level, we must implement a protective system. True capitalism has proved to be the only working compromise in this regard.

By creating competition, capitalism and a free-market economy ensure that people have common interests and use their greed, pride, and thirst for power constructively. Of course, this would only limit and restrict our destructive potential, rather than trying to suppress our nature as socialism and communism do aggressively.

The problem with socialism and Marxism is that they never had a Nuremberg trial process as the Nazis and the extreme right had. No one has tried to define where the limits should lie in this utopia of egalitarianism and regulation. We urgently need a trial of this dangerous mental cancer. This well-intended but so malefic ideology has proven to be just as devastating over and over in different forms, at different times, and in different circumstances.

Our present vocabulary associates terms like "fascist" or "Nazi" with an extreme, dangerous, and right-wing ideology. Yet there is no equivalent term denoting the extreme left.

Interestingly, socialism and communism, concepts that reside at the extreme left of the political spectrum, are often viewed as unproblematic. Even worse, they're sometimes even considered to be trendy in our evolving societal norms. The global reset propaganda of the World Economic Forum falls in this category.

Nowadays, this discrepancy—which arises from a deficiency in cultural and historical awareness—is carefully maintained and supported in most colleges and universities. Sadly, this propaganda leaves most uninformed or misinformed about the severe brutality and destruction that communist regimes have produced in the past—damage that has greatly surpassed the cruelty and devastation caused by fascism. We badly need a communism trial. This should be a trial similar to the Nuremberg trial but aimed at communism. This would serve to define and prosecute the left ideology in a manner analogous to how the Nuremberg trial addressed the right ideology.

The United States has the most proven system designed to deal with human nature.

Throughout history, it has become evident that individuals who acquire more power often tend to misuse it. This pattern arises because, fundamentally, we are still driven by our primal instincts as animals, and our consciousness alone is insufficient to prevent the abuse of power. Not even spirituality or the fear of God can control our natural abusive impulses. However, men who feared nothing, not even God, demonstrated the worst cases of abuse of power.

Consider the destruction caused by Mao, Stalin, and Hitler. Throughout human history, and even in modern times, when nations and organizations acquire sufficient power, that power is almost always abused. Everyone expanded as much as possible, from the Roman Empire to the British Empire to Hitler and the USSR. During the era when tribal communities were prevalent, which ended just a few centuries ago for a large portion of the world, a recurring pattern emerged. Because of the absence of established laws or protective pacts, this certain scenario unfolded: If one community grew significantly stronger than others, it frequently resulted in its weaker neighbors' exploitation, enslavement, or extermination. Unfortunately, this pattern still occurs in certain remote areas today.

Today Russia and China are taking enlargement measures. Consider Hong Kong and the seas surrounding various areas with a Chinese presence. Or, in the case of Russia, look at Georgia and Ukraine. The only exception so far is the United States. For a long time, the U.S. was the sole superpower that could easily occupy multiple additional territories, but it did not even touch Cuba.

Evidently, if the U.S. had not dominated the seas, trading, and commerce by having widespread military bases, submarines, and aircraft carriers, China, Russia, or another superpower would have done it. And history clearly shows which alternative is better.

A better, "ideal" alternative—in which there is no dominance, conflict, and self-interest, in which everybody would be happy and treated fairly—would be completely utopic, possible only in the dream of the naive.

The U.S. system had proven to be a constructive, positive, and good system through the remarkable examples of Japan, South Korea, and West Germany. After World War II, the Americans imposed their democratic, free market, capitalist system on the occupied territories for at least ten years. This resulted in great prosperity, freedom, and stability. It's easy to observe that American democracy and capitalism are superior systems. This can especially be concluded when comparing the same nations split into West and East Germany and South and North Korea. The half of the country that introduced the socialism-communism system proved inferior with disastrous results, ending in reduced prosperity and freedom—and in North Korea's case, extreme totalitarianism.

A similar situation is happening today in South Africa. Things have significantly worsened each year after the British left. The English brought democracy and significant economic improvements, leading the country to stability and prosperity.

After British control was transferred to China, Hong Kong has been deteriorating economically, culturally, and especially socially, with a significant loss of freedom of speech.

In the past few decades, though, when the U.S. temporarily occupied other countries, unfortunately, due to Washington's new policies of "noninterference," part of the new culture that has plagued Western civilization for the past few decades, it did not impose the democratic system with capitalist markets, separation of powers, free elections, or free speech anymore.

Therefore, those countries could not prosper and even radicalize further because they maintained their old systems.

Consider, for example, the chaos in Afghanistan, Libya, Syria, and Iraq. Liberating a totalitarian regime from a dictator is not enough. The vacuum of power left needs to be replaced with something good, stable, and reliable. If we don't impose our proven democratic system, we better not interfere.

These examples show the disastrous effect of the new wave of rich, overnight corrupted politicians thriving in an unconstitutional permanent Washington. Add to it the new culture, in which the true values of the Western culture are thrown away in exchange for utopian, equalitarian, "anti-imperialist," "anti-racist," anti-capitalist, and globalist philosophies, with strong Marxist influences. This urgently needs to be stopped before it's too late. All politicians should be limited to two terms or eight years of active involvement, and extensions up to another term should be limited and only approved under exceptional circumstances through special elections.

The United States represents the pyramid's pinnacle in human society's evolution. It is the only large country and system that has never had a dictator, emperor, or other radical movement. Why? Because the Founding Fathers, realizing how destructive humans are, found an imperfect yet proven solution: the Constitution of the United States. This integral document prevents the centralization of power. It limits and splits the powers of a single individual as well as the powers of various groups and organizations with the same interests. This division of powers and responsibilities does not eliminate conflicts but limits and balances them.

The size of the middle class has been shrinking significantly. The middle class is an accurate measure of a country's freedom and prosperity.

The U.S. Constitution and legal system allowed and encouraged Americans to create the most extensive and robust middle class in history. I believe that the size and wealth of the middle class are directly correlated with the country's prosperity as a whole, including that of people with low incomes. The middle class that has shrunk the most is represented largely by small and medium-sized businesses such as restaurants, law firms, clinics, auto repair shops, and so on.

If we look at all totalitarian regimes, the middle class is either small or non-existent. A regime that abuses power has only a high class and a low class. We need a robust middle class to achieve balance and prevent abuse by the upper classes, especially since they contain so much powerful influence over the state and the government.

History has repeatedly shown that the lower classes can be easily manipulated and brainwashed. When conditions go to extremes, they can fight back through revolt. As we know, voters' opinions can be easily manipulated through TV and social media by the few who create and contain the information. It's much harder to manipulate the middle class, as it has more involvement and significantly greater political power and influence.

Regrettably, over the past few decades, there has been a notable decline in the size of the middle class in the United States, accompanied by a significant shift in power toward the upper class. This shift is evident in the escalating number of billionaires who have experienced substantial financial growth and wield considerable political influence. Consequently, there is a growing tendency among these billionaires to prioritize their personal interests over the nation's. And now they are all forced to align with the new global interest led by the World Economic Forum. We need more brave entrepreneurs like Elon Musk, who has the courage to oppose it. He gave us one of the few free-speech social platforms, X (the old, corrupted Twitter) restructured and cleaned from government control.

The increasing burden of excessive regulations imposed by the government has posed significant challenges, particularly for small businesses, resulting in the unfortunate closure of many of them. Unlike larger corporations, which can navigate regulatory requirements more adeptly, these small enterprises often struggle to comply. Furthermore, concerns arise as many multibillion-dollar companies extend their influence through lobbying, corruption, and the acquisition of competitors and adversaries. As a result, individuals in the lower and middle classes often suffer from these circumstances.

Consider the behavior of major American airline companies, which often exhibit a lack of regard and mistreatment towards their customers. There are frequent instances of flight and seat changes or cancellations that often leave passengers with no choice but to settle for alternative options that are typically inferior or even unacceptable. These companies prioritize quantity over quality, resulting in compromised customer experiences.

Furthermore, a concerning general trend is emerging across various sectors, encompassing insurance, software, social media, and banking, where large corporations exploit their power by increasing costs, taking shortcuts, and diminishing overall service quality.

Here's what's scary: These companies can pull this off without consequences. Why? Because the old, good, free market, competition-based mechanisms for countering abuse and maintaining quality have been hacked and destroyed. In many industries, there is a behind-the-scenes monopoly that has been forming as part of the general globalization policies led by centralized, global financial institutions. Nothing can stop them anymore.

The abuse of those in power has taken a more subtle but broader form in recent decades.

The United States has undoubtedly leveraged its position of power to further its interests. This is particularly evident in the unfolding stories of abuse of power by influential groups, especially within the military and pharmaceutical complexes.

These industries are known for their profit-driven motives and desire for control, a fact that is increasingly being revealed. Many conspiracy theories have amazingly proven to be true. The military industry, following a global agenda, is often implicated in initiating or exacerbating conflicts elsewhere in the world to secure lucrative contracts and assert geopolitical and economic dominance.

Similarly, the pharmaceutical industry has been scrutinized for practices such as overpricing vital medications, pushing vaccines, and lobbying for legislation that serves their profit margins at the cost of public health. Both industries extend their influence worldwide, often resulting in a global impact.

The question is where reasonableness stops, and abuse starts. Obviously, morality is not enough. The systems already in place designed to control these abuses are definitely not working.

The ideal arbitrator does not exist.

In an ideal world, there would be an arbitrator—an all-knowing and wise alien power who would oversee these conflicts and abuses and minimize or eliminate them. (Yes, I am joking.) But even if this did exist, who would stop the alien power from taking advantage of the less powerful? Well, because they wouldn't be human, perhaps they wouldn't abuse their power. Maybe they wouldn't have a destructive nature, judging by the fact that humanity advanced so much, possibly with their help. However, they are not getting involved directly, so far, so we have no better alternative than a constitution like the U.S. Constitution.

Time has proven this to be the best option for protecting the lives and liberties of everyone.

If aliens are indeed present here, even though they are vastly superior in knowledge and technology to human achievements, they must still be fascinated by the nature's intelligence of this planet, as is designed by our Creator, who is the same Creator as theirs. Their actions could still be viewed with respect to their Creator's purpose for them. They would also be subject to the entropic perspective, which is the direction of the actions toward creation or destruction, toward their higher purpose or away from it.

The U.S. Constitution is the only proven, available solution, but it needs to be complemented at the individual-personal level.

America's Bill of Rights and the structure of power distribution detailed in the Constitution primarily serve to safeguard individuals from each other. However, these do not have the capacity to shield a person from their own actions or decisions. That obligation relies on personal elements such as spirituality, religious beliefs, and scientific understanding, specifically in the fields of psychology and psychiatry. History and wisdom have demonstrated that attempts to control individual behavior led to misuse and exploitation; thus, no organization should endeavor such regulation.

Only in extreme circumstances, such as someone contemplating suicide, should that individual be involuntarily detained (per the Baker Act), but these cases are the exception, not the rule.

Due to our primitive animal nature, totally free men tend to be destructive and dangerous. We respond effectively to fear of *immediate* consequences and less effectively to *remote* consequences; finding this middle ground between freedom and fear, however, is difficult. So far, the original U.S. system is the best compromise.

What is complete freedom? We know how people behave when they are enabled with total freedom. Most of the time, they grow into monsters. If change and radicalization are introduced slowly, the effects are less obvious, better tolerated, and more likely to succeed. If this happens to people with power, it creates humanitarian disasters.

Here are two significant cases:

Mao Zedong's Cultural Revolution in China: Mao's regime is an example of unchecked power leading to atrocities. Mao introduced radical changes gradually, starting with land reform and culminating in the Cultural Revolution. This decade-long period was marked by purges, public humiliation, and violent persecution, resulting in millions of deaths.

Joseph Stalin's USSR: Stalin gradually centralized power and imposed severe restrictions on personal freedoms. Under the guise of industrialization and collectivization, millions of people were purged, executed, or sent to labor camps known as gulags. The regime's oppressive policies were introduced slowly, making them less noticeable until they had become deeply entrenched.

If you need more convincing, watch the movie "The Experiment," made after a real scientific psychological study in 1971 at Stanford University. In it, average students were split into two groups, guards and prisoners, in a two-week mock prison experiment. It demonstrates how, at a small scale, at the individual level, an average person, if enabled, can quickly transform into a monster.

A new global order

A new, utopian governmental solution—designed to address the challenges of modern society and minimize human suffering—plans to transition everyone into a virtual world with the help of artificial intelligence (AI). This vision sets a common objective, a worldwide initiative involving all nations. This objective encourages adherence to a universal system of rules and protections, which includes health and educational programs.

For instance, if all cars were fully automated and driven by AI, it would drastically reduce car accidents. This single adjustment is significant, considering there are 30,000 to 40,000 fatalities annually and several million disabilities resulting from road accidents in the United States alone.

Sure, this transformation promises enhanced safety, but it would also relinquish our ability to personally drive a car. Instead, we would be totally dependent.

Gradually acquainting society with the benefits and conveniences of an AI-guided virtual world could promote safety, as many resultant consequences would be virtual rather than real. However, the real, non-virtual impact on each individual is significant and remains unknown and likely disastrous.

This "progress" comes at the cost of our freedom. As safety and freedom often move in opposing directions, striking a balance is necessary. Yet, suppose the power to determine this balance resides solely with those in authority. In that case, it is inevitable, given human nature and the lessons of history, that this power will be exploited to their advantage, towards safety and control and away from freedom. As Benjamin Franklin famously said:

"Those who would give up essential Liberty, to purchase a little temporary Safety, deserve neither Liberty nor Safety."

Another obvious danger is coming directly from AI. Artificial intelligence will discourage and destroy our creativity. All artists and creators are in danger, as AI can easily create art in all forms and shapes, from music to paintings to movies and books.

We may benefit from developing an AW (artificial wisdom) rather than AI. AI is focused on efficiency and comfort, while AW would focus on applying old wisdom to achieve higher purposes and give meaning to our lives, as I described in earlier chapters. There is a contradiction in terms here as wisdom comes from God the creator, and we could not call it artificial. The intelligence and wisdom of nature that made life thrive and created humanity, the tip of the pyramid here on Earth, is far more advanced than any AI could ever achieve. We have a long way to go before we can comprehend nature, but that is where artificial intelligence and artificial wisdom should get their resources. What we know now is barely scratching its surface.

And what would stop AI from eventually turning against humankind?

Thanks to technological automation, the manufacturing industry has shrunk dramatically from fifty years ago.

In contemporary Western societies, the primary means of earning a livelihood mostly entails providing services to others. However, as we approach a future where AI and humanoid robots are widely accepted, there will be a significant transformation in this employment landscape. These technological advancements, aimed at offering superior convenience and reliability, are gradually being adopted and will likely render most traditional service roles obsolete.

Our 21st-century culture is increasingly promoting the values of comfort, convenience, and safety at the expense of independence, challenges, and freedom. Consequently, the only way for us to obtain the essential needs of life (purpose, satisfaction of achievement, and connecting) while staying "safe" is to move into this virtual world.

This new Great Reset Initiative creates the environment for this to occur. This will minimize conflict and suffering because a virtual world allows us to take risks without facing the consequences. This also minimizes our destruction to this planet, reducing pollution and waste—a perfect agenda. As is the promise: We will own nothing, probably not even our own body, but live in peace, free from challenges, stress and conflicts. Like in "The Matrix" movie, we would all live in a safe bubble. Sounds ideal, right?

But this is another utopia like Marx's of 150 years ago. The main problem with these philosophies is that they ignore human nature. There will always be people who crave more freedom and diversity, as nature's laws cannot be bent. People will question circumstances and want to be free and make changes. It also goes against natural law, as we need natural challenges to develop, grow, and survive. The virtual challenges, at least for an extended period, would not match the natural ones.

As the new world order is formed by introducing a new centralized and universal culture, it will continue to destroy the old cultural and spiritual values, such as the family unit and Christianity or other major religions (factors that are the core of a stable society).

To make this possible, the people behind this global reset plan need to create chaos and crisis, as radical changes are difficult to introduce in a stable, happy society.

It should be called the new global *dis*order instead. Population aging is one of the consequences of this new culture. In this new culture, the family is no longer central to society. Hence, people are less concerned with having children and more with the single's freedom or multiple opportunities. To compensate for and resolve the aging problem in Europe, a policy to accept immigrants from different cultures and religions has been applied for the past fifteen to twenty years.

The problem is that most of these new immigrants do not integrate into the host country's Christian culture. This creates fragmentation and separation and can ultimately result in chaos. As previously discussed, a functioning system requires order, common purposes, and values.

Western Europe has also seen a dramatic decline in the proportion of the population that would be considered Christian, primarily due to cultural changes as well as massive immigration.

The Christian church is a primary culprit for these cultural changes in Western civilization. Starting over 100 years ago, the Christian church in the U.S. also shifted its focus and responsibility from influencing the country's culture to influencing the individual's life alone. This is highly inefficient as it is much more efficient to influence people through culture than individually.

The resulting rising rates of divorce and single parenthood are associated with poverty, lack of education, and increased crime rates, beginning in adolescence. Instilling the value of family and lowering the divorce rate is one of the most important solutions to move any country back in the right direction.

This illustrates the consequence of prioritizing human uneducated construct over nature's design. In many contemporary Western cultures, there's an emphasis on absolute gender equality. This often promotes the idea of an independent woman who is less inclined towards starting a family because of career and financial responsibilities. Such a shift can devalue the traditional family structure, resulting in a rise in single individuals and single-parent households. This trend reduces birth rates, leading to an aging population and potential depopulation. Additionally, these changes can bring about financial, psychological, and social challenges.

The young new generations, including educated ones, are doomed. Returning to our roots is the solution. Here is a possible scenario:

For the past forty years, at least, Western civilizations have witnessed a massive migration of young people from the countryside and rural areas to the big cities. This migration also contributed to the decline in the modern cultural value of family. A family-oriented culture is essential for survival in rural areas and less so in large cities. But over the years, college graduates have been paid less and less, making it more difficult to find jobs that match their qualifications. For the younger generations, after graduation from college, it's becoming more and more difficult to thrive and even to survive.

This, combined with a looming deep recession—with rising prices for everything from real estate and rent to cars, energy, and groceries—will force the younger population to return to rural areas. Living in the countryside makes people more self-sufficient and family oriented. They are more likely to survive an economic crisis. This also reduces their dependence on states and other centralized powers, a dependence that has expanded dramatically in recent years as part of the new globalization trend.

In the longer term, as automatization and AI are going to take over even the last job field that needs people—the services—most of the population will have no job and nothing to do. The solution is to return to our design, move to the countryside and live in nature as farmers with clean, modern technology. The physical work will be much less demanding than in the past, as farming machines will be available to rent or purchase. Fishing and hunting will be resumed. Raising farm animals will be essential. It will provide a higher quality of nutrition and health.

A high-speed train network will provide individuals access to the big cities and other entertainment areas. We will also stay well connected, virtually, with friends and other family members.

Staying clustered in big cities and suburbs will continue to make us unhealthy and dependent on the government and the global regulation system, which has proven very incompetent and harmful.

The expansion of authorities' powers in the past decades accelerated during the COVID-19 pandemic.

With the help of most media, for at least the past forty to fifty years, the elites have been working to brainwash the population, to make it believe, first, in the '70s and '80s, that there was going to be an ice age by, the end of the 20th century, then that we're going to run out of fossil fuel by the year 2000. Lately, they changed the narrative to global warming's imminent dangers, and most recently, the COVID-19 and other looming pandemic crises, requiring global control and newly enforced central regulations.

What happened with the COVID pandemic proves that the corruption of large corporations, interfering in people's lives alongside the government for their own benefit, has reached unprecedented levels in modern Western civilization.

The horrific abuses in the name of COVID in China do not surprise me, as their president and the authorities had already wielded an unprecedented amount of authoritarian power.

As evidence mounts that governments' various approaches to combating the coronavirus pandemic have failed, people have lost faith in science and medicine, creating a vacuum of trust. This will lead to chaos as there are fewer reliable sources of information. And without a reliable check system, people will believe and follow what is convenient or available and become more susceptible to manipulation.

One might reasonably argue that, in 2020, little was known about what was happening, so extreme measures became justified in the crisis. After the crisis dissipated in 2022 and more information became available, the government and pharmaceutical corporations continued to push the vaccine, even for children, pregnant women, and healthy young adults, for no reasonable justification. Even more concerning is that it was not a mere imposition but rather an utterly unjust mandate that violated fundamental human rights.

In 2022, COVID was no longer a significant threat—not any more than the flu was. So why mandate experimental injectable vaccination of young, healthy individuals? Why ignore the data showing that its benefits and side effects are unacceptable and not what we initially expected?

This phenomenon has occurred many times throughout history. At some point, even if society is faced with the truth and with evidence, many will refuse to admit the mistake and back down.

It is human nature to be driven by pride, shame, and fear. More frightening is that these abuses by authorities occur almost globally.

What even more amazes me is seeing how most people, including medical personnel and doctors, readily accepted and trusted the system even two years later, despite ample evidence to the contrary.

This results from the new culture created in schools and universities over the past thirty-plus years, leading to a shift from traditional values. I don't want to describe in detail the amount of cheating and wrongdoing that occurred during this pandemic. This example of power abuse shows that human nature has not changed, and that history can and will repeat itself.

The crisis caused by the pandemic has significantly escalated conflicts between individuals and authorities, pushing the entire society toward the last phase of the Tytler cycle—the Dependence into the Bondage stage.

The cultural differences between the United States and Europe and their significant consequences on individual well-being.

The American culture puts significant peer pressure on financial gain and success on Americans. The American dream got distorted and expanded from having a big house, a large family, and multiple cars to becoming rich overnight. The amazing success of some individuals who became millionaires overnight, enabled by social media and advancing technology, created this new dream for younger generations. We are all now potential millionaires, and our jobs are just a fill-in until it happens. It is the American capitalism, constitution, and financial system that make this possible.

This is very unlikely to happen in other countries as they have a more socialistic model of economy and society, having much less to offer to the individual. As a result, in Western European countries, people are focused more on relaxing and having free time, and there is less obsession with money and the materialistic aspect of life. The average time off and vacations in Western Europe is almost triple that of American counterparts.

The more you work, the more you gain—this motto is often valid in the United States. It enables our natural greed: the more you have, the more you want. This function works well in the United States but not so much in Western Europe or the rest of the world. This is why the United States has led the world in innovation and development.

This is good for the successful ones and society as a whole, for the advancement of humanity, but not so much for most individuals. For most Americans, this financial and social success remains just a dream, and they live their entire life under this cultural and psychological pressure focused on materialism. It also makes quantity more important than quality.

This may be one reason why the quality of foods in the United States is so low compared with Western European countries. It is well known that Americans traveling to Europe, even if they abuse food, usually would not gain significant weight and would see an improvement in chronic digestive symptoms and other illnesses. There are many agricultural products made in the United States that are banned in Europe due to too much human intervention, from food processing, chemical additives, and contamination to genetic modifications. The taste of most groceries is significantly better in most European countries. It fades away every year in large American grocery stores as the soil used to grow foods on a large scale is getting poorer in minerals and higher in unhealthy artificial pesticides and fertilizers.

Gabriel is a patient of mine in his late forties who, a few years ago, developed a progressive, severe, debilitating neurological condition manifested in double vision, significant balance impairment, and muscle weakness, among multiple other neurological symptoms. He had seen many specialists and had extensive workups that only identified damages in his cerebellum but not the cause. Gabriel tried various treatments without any success. Significantly, he reported that the severity of his symptoms varies considerably depending on his diet and lifestyle. If he fasts or eats a low-carb diet, he feels better. He cannot function for hours and even days when he makes mistakes, like eating fast food or pizza. Most types of grains worsen his condition.

He recently spent three months visiting the Philippines and stayed with his wife's sister. There, he ate mostly cooked food made by his sister-in-law. He made significant improvements in his vision and balance. He said he had at least a sixty to seventy percent improvement compared with when he left the United States. He was able to ride a bike and play pool for the first time in almost a decade. Sadly, a few days after he returned to the United States, he was back the way he had left here, with a full return of all his neurological symptoms. Yet his home diet in Florida was similar to his diet in the Philippines—in fact, even more aggressive with carbs restrictions.

So again, quantity over quality is more easily accepted in the United States culture but has a detrimental effect on our health and well-being. This is reflected in the data that shows that Americans, in general, suffer more from chronic diseases and have higher adult mortality and infant mortality rates than most Western European countries. This is even though significantly more money is spent on healthcare per capita in the United States.

Intelligence alone is not enough to protect us from our self-destructive nature.

What restrictions are needed to limit the destruction a free man can wreak upon others and himself? Is fear enough to control? Is morality enough, and is spirituality necessary?

Morality is rooted in natural countertransference when we consciously or subconsciously project ourselves into another person's place to see and feel from their perspective. Stealing and cheating are immoral. It is *moral* to help your neighbor or to protect the weak.

Loving your enemies, loving unconditionally without expecting reciprocity, and deferring judgment are beyond morality. These don't come easy or naturally; they are spiritual in nature.

How do young adults know what is good for them? Most likely, they don't learn these things on their own; they shouldn't need to. Home education and school help young people avoid unnecessary struggle and harm, but unfortunately, this is usually not enough. Young people mostly learn through their own experiences rather than those of others, and not always from good experiences. Negative experiential learning does not need to occur.

Can we skip this entirely and escape the pain and suffering? No, but fortunately, much unnecessary suffering can be avoided by acting on wisdom.

We can add new wisdom by applying ancient wisdom and spirituality together with insights from the modern discoveries of science and technology. And yet we must still accept that human nature has not changed and often causes self-inflicted harm.

Unfortunately, today's modern psychology and psychiatry are far from being able to understand and control the human mind and behavior.

Intelligence and wisdom can go in opposite directions. While intelligence is purely human and can be easily used for rationalization to satisfy primal unconscious impulses, wisdom comes primarily through accumulated experiences and revelation and is spiritual.

Intelligence without wisdom is dangerous!

Science creates and accumulates knowledge but cannot and should not interpret and apply it at a large scale by itself. Scientism is a new, dangerous ideology.

Unfortunately, today, there is a widespread and growing belief that science can understand and solve most, if not all, of humanity's social and individual problems. This phenomenon is a new ideology, part of the modern culture, called *scientism*.

In the past few decades, scientism has been extensively taught in schools and colleges. It is an ideology that holds that science is the sole or primary source of knowledge. It enforces that scientific methods and principles can be applied to all areas of inquiry, including those traditionally addressed by philosophy, ethics, religion, and other disciplines. It emphasizes the idea that empirical evidence and scientific reasoning are the only valid means of understanding the world and making informed decisions.

The believers in scientism argue that scientific knowledge is superior to other forms of knowledge because it is based on empirical evidence, rigorous observation, experimentation, and logical analysis. They often view science as a unified and self-correcting method that can provide answers to all questions and address all human concerns. This cannot be further from the truth. The ability of science to explore different system details and understand mechanisms of functioning does not extend, as many want to believe, into understanding the purposes of various systems as a whole. To attain a global perspective, the integration of numerous other disciplines—philosophy, geopolitics, history, and particularly spirituality—is essential.

Healthy fear protects us from immediate as well as distant consequences.

Wisdom is the final solution. It teaches us to stop living in a mostly reactive state, one that is driven by primitive impulses. Instead, we must react to wisdom's insights as strongly as we respond to threats or joy.

In other words, we must live by solid principles, character, and virtue.

Phillips Brooks, renowned American minister, offers this sound advice:

> *"Someday, in the years to come, you will be wrestling with the great temptation or trembling under the great sorrow of your life. But the real struggle is here, now... Now it is being decided whether, in the day of your supreme sorrow or temptation, you shall miserably fail or gloriously conquer. The character cannot be made except by a steady, long, continued process."*

Let us learn to fear the warnings of old wisdom. The Bible reveals this in Proverbs 9:10: *"The fear of God is the beginning of wisdom."*

Unfortunately, most of us do not develop fears over an idea or abstract concepts unless there is an obvious motive or immediate threat. We usually need to experience the consequence before we react. It's important to respond early, rather than live in denial until serious and sometimes irreversible repercussions occur.

Which outcome should we prefer: to hold faith in a God who is not certain to exist or to reject belief in a God who actually *does* exist?

Everything we do or don't do has consequences. As a popular quote states:

"There are in nature neither rewards nor punishments—there are consequences."

In this regard, our reality is quite unfortunate. We are victims of the nature of the *human mind.*

Having lived for over twenty-five years in Romania, which had been enduring over forty years of communism, I learned how corrupt people can become.

In its worst years, most Romanian workers cut corners and provided low-quality services due to a lack of personal interest. The government controlled everything. For over ninety percent of the population, it was clear that the government was an enemy of the people. The same was true for most countries in the Eastern Bloc.

I never thought I would witness it almost as bad here in the United States, except that the U.S. government is still considered good by many. Just like in Romania, in America, the quality of services has decreased significantly—particularly since COVID began. Lately, people can afford to cut corners without experiencing any consequences and have considerably less personal interest or concern over the quality of services they provide.

How can businesses and workers get away with this? All they need is an excuse. For instance, "It is because of COVID," or, "If I don't work, then I get paid by the government through unemployment anyway." People have also said, "If I lose this job, then I can easily find another one since the demand is so high due to the economic crisis."

What happened to our education and principles? What happened to our fear of consequences? Not having a healthy fear of losing your job or income is destructive. This is more prominent among the employees of large companies, as those are becoming more monopolies, immune to competition, as described earlier in the chapter. The pandemic has led to a crisis of quality jobs, also affecting the middle class and small businesses.

Unfortunately, fear is, and always will be, the dominant driving force here. We behave primitively. A look at companies of different sizes reveals a broad spectrum of quality of care and services. If small businesses or local businesses do not provide good quality services, customers will not return, and many businesses may disappear and lose everything. Large chains, on the other hand, are protected by their size. So, unless a rigorous training and enforcement system is in place, the quality of service can remain poor. They have different values.

The state, being the largest "company," provides the worst possible environment for its employees, as they have no reason to be concerned about the consequences of lousy work (other than potential reprimands from a supervisor).

The younger generation, in particular, seems to have different values. It appears increasingly uninterested in producing quality work and services. Part of this is due to social media. After all, everyone is a potential millionaire or celebrity in the social media virtual world—so, at home, people feel used because, in the real world, they must work and serve others.

The domino effect.

We are part of a complex picture over which we have little control, which is one of the main reasons life is unfair. Everything that occurs comes from much more than we can comprehend. It results from a complex chain of events and facts, like a set of dominoes falling.

The influences we experience come from different directions and levels: external factors such as our environment, social setting, and geography; internal genetic factors that intermingle with external factors; and influences from our present life, including our habits and environment.

Everything is how it's supposed to be because each event has the power and merit to exist.

Every occurrence is a consequence of a complex chain of mostly unavoidable events. For example, a death or injury resulting from a car accident could be traced back to a very intricate chain of events that began long before the accident and might have originated years or even generations before.

Suffering is often unavoidable and natural—the origin of evil, pain, and suffering.

The propensity of our world for destruction and chaos is not necessarily evil; it is, in fact, the norm. The exception is the unique constructive forces that come from God's design. To maintain order and complexity, work is required. A relationship without work will disintegrate, and anything that doesn't demand constructive effort will deteriorate quickly. That's not a bad thing. It is simply the way the universe is built. Yes, there is evil in this world—but most of it is due to man's wrongdoing. Evil almost always acts on Earth through human weaknesses and destructive propensity, which is easily observed in most religious scriptures.

Many people ask how God is good when so much suffering happens in this world.

Suffering is rooted in the very nature of existence and manifestation. It is the price of freedom and independence, the cost of unlimited expression and infinite diversity. When God, the Creator, made a conscious mind and its freedom to choose, this unavoidably resulted in conflict. There are unavoidable circumstances in which only one can prevail, leading to rivalry. Conflict and competition are significant causes of distress and suffering. As the saying goes, *"The winner takes it all."*

In biblical terms, when God created the angels, they obeyed and followed Him faithfully. However, God gave them freedom of choice. This became the source of conflict when some of them naturally opposed each other and eventually rebelled against God Himself. This is the price of independence and freedom, and it is how independent angels became evil by opposing God, resulting in the emergence of the devil and demons in the spiritual world.

The same thing happened in the material world when Adam and Eve were given freedom and independence. Before that, with God's permission, they lived in peace without conflicts, following a perfect order. By giving them a conscious mind and the power to choose, by making them in His image, God created man. Conflicts and disagreements were unavoidable as the independent decisions one individual makes won't always align with the choices of others.

And unfortunately, this reality multiplied and propagated as life was made that way: to change, self-evolve, and grow through experimentation and challenge. We inherit prior conflicts in our genes since human existence.

Why did God allow harmful past experiences to be transmitted and disseminated? This is because the whole system relies on experiences. We cannot value the good without experiencing the bad, as these two are inherently linked. Our lives revolve around comparisons. Challenges bring about suffering. Without challenges, there is no growth or learning. Consequently, there would be no evolution, advancement, or freedom. Darwin called this "survival of the fittest" the backbone of evolution.

"If it does not challenge you, it doesn't change you."
—Fred DeVito, author and fitness trainer

A Christian perspective: the relationship between man and God.

God wants us to discover everything for ourselves. Being created in His image, He wants us to be free and independent so that we can be exposed to everything and grow on our own through challenges and failures. At least until we are ready to receive the revelation of our Creator. Our life on Earth, through our body and mind, provides us and our souls with an opportunity to draw closer to the Creator, relate to Him, and become more like Him. This may be our souls' only opportunity, as we are represented in eternity by our souls.

In other words, God's purpose for us is to discover and appreciate Him and His creation and return to Him by our own will and choice. That is called faith. He also desires that we follow Him out of love and appreciation, not just by self-interest, fear, or obedience. Moreover, He wants us not only to resemble Him but also to act like Him, to be creative and constructive, and to combat destructive forces.

As part of our relationship with God, He wants us to experience and appreciate His creation and work, encouraging us to imitate Him. He desires to share His love, hopes, goals, and purposes. He appreciates complexities, challenges, and even complications. In fact, this is part of His overall plan for this universe to diversify and expand in its expressions.

Advances in technology have vastly improved access to information and facilitated communication between different peoples and cultures. It has given us more opportunities to be creative and constructive. The full spectrum of human qualities and imperfections has been exposed and learned like never before.

Speaking about being grateful for what we have in the 21st century, in the past fifty to a hundred years, a middle-class individual could afford a life that only a few wealthy people could afford just a couple of hundred years ago. This is due to the advancements in technology, science, and culture. We suffer much less in terms of necessary suffering. But are we happier? Do we actually suffer less overall? A few hundred years ago, people had no choice regarding the pain in their lives. But today, much of the pain we experience is unnecessary and self-induced.

Today, as always, we experience the consequences of both our ancestors' and our own choices. God is good because He created life, maintains order in a chaotic universe, and prevents man from complete self-destruction. He helps man to evolve, thrive, and prosper by giving us free choice, consciousness, awareness, and constant opportunities to know and relate to Him. Christians believe that spiritual knowledge of and relationship with God is their only way to escape the long-term consequences of their inherently destructive human nature.

Why is God so abstract and unseen? If humans had a direct relationship with God similar to normal human relationships, sooner or later—because of our nature—we would end up abusing God with our judgments, requests, needs, and fears. He must remain untouchable. Just consider, for example, what we did to Jesus.

From Christianity's perspective, we are born with an enormous debt inherited from Adam and Eve, and this debt has been passed on through their descendants. We are born with significant liability, but we have a chance to be absolved by transferring this debt to Jesus, who offered to take it upon himself and redeem man from his own wrongdoings.

The Bible is clear: we cannot rectify past mistakes and sins. We also cannot carry and solve our burdens. But we don't need to because that is why Jesus came on Earth, to take it all upon Himself and to do justice for all. The only thing we need to do is to believe in and follow Him. There is no need to perform to be competitive or successful; we only need faith.

> *"For by grace you have been saved through faith; and that not of yourselves, it is the gift of God; not as a result of works, so that no one may boast"* (Ephesians 2:8-9, New American Standard Bible).

The important constructive role of Christianity in the development of modern society.

Christianity is an open and nondiscriminatory religion that has contributed significantly to the evolution of our civilization.

Christianity is unique in that it's the only major philosophy that treats women at the same level as men and accepts the separation of powers in the state.

Any abuses committed in the name of Christianity do not come from its philosophy but rather from our natural tendency to abuse power when given the opportunity. In fact, the main reason that Christianity accepted the separation of powers in the state was to prevent the abuse committed by individuals in power.

Christianity is not radical at its core because it preaches forgiveness over justice and makes all equal before God. Christian societies have been the foundation of Western societies, contributing to the advancement of technology, science, culture, and civilization.

Jesus encouraged the separation of the powers in the state, which was later accepted by Christianity. This was one of the main reasons why science and technology flourished. It is also how Western culture and civilization can coexist with spirituality and science. God wanted us to multiply and thrive, and this prosperity would not have been possible without technological advances.

If we were to live forever on Earth, we would continuously accumulate the consequences of our actions on top of those of our ancestors. This would be an unbearable burden. Canceling this "debt" and achieving freedom from these consequences is not possible here on Earth. According to Christianity, it is possible only after we die, as we continue to live through our souls. Christians call the process of canceling the consequences we were supposed to pay "propitiation," as Jesus paid our debt.

The limits of our mind and thought.

The way we are designed reveals our limitations. Our thinking is linear in time and space, which limits and prevents us from understanding unresolved concepts like infinity. We cannot understand who created the Creator because we cannot comprehend what lies beyond the universe, beyond the *end of the end,* or answer the popular question: "Which came first, the chicken or the egg?" In doing so, we acknowledge our limitations and recognize that the Creator is more powerful than creation itself.

Another example is the antinomy of free choice and destiny. How can they both be true at the same time?

We can imagine the existence of other dimensions, but we cannot directly access or explore them. We can only be aware of them and recognize our own limitations.

"We can know only that we know nothing. And that is the highest degree of human wisdom."

—Leo Tolstoy

Based on mathematical and scientific principles, theoretically, anything could occur given infinite time and space. For instance, the probability of an elephant materializing in Antarctica is not zero but extremely minute. Theoretically, this could happen within the boundless expanse of time and space. Yet, in reality, it's impossible because the universe is structured with intention and purpose, not solely driven by physics and mathematical laws. There exist unseen regulations governing all things, rules beyond our comprehension. These laws prevent occurrences that, while theoretically possible in a mathematical sense, are otherwise irrational.

A domino-like model of the universe.

For simplification and better illustration, here's an analogy: The entire system of the world we know, with all its subsystems, can be compared to a predesigned yet not manifested complex and complicated domino system. The tracks of the domino system were created with the purpose of manifestation and diversification. In Latin, *domino* means master, which reveals the Creator of this domino system, our Creator. Manifestation, in this sense, means that the system both exists and transforms.

This complex, intricate, predesigned domino system has various (but still limited) possible outcomes, including local life situations for all of us.

The domino patterns are created and, in action, constantly advancing. Each life with its events represents a "miniature domino" in the extensive domino system—one small piece of the whole with a limited outcome, as it must align with the higher purpose, just as subsystems serve higher systems. Nevertheless, each part of the domino is essential, as a missing piece may profoundly alter the pattern. In this domino design, random alternate pathways are possible, but only within the limits of its creation.

Everything is pre-created but not yet manifested. Everything is predestined but not yet demonstrated. And, of course, the Creator can intervene and change the pattern.

This is how God can be both Creator and the highest Purpose, the pinnacle of the purpose hierarchy, as He created everything from the beginning, yet each intricate detail is only revealed in its time. The Bible suggests this concept:

"I make known the end from the beginning, from ancient times, what is still to come. I say, 'My purpose will stand, and I will do all that I please."

—Isaiah 46:10

"I am the Alpha and the Omega, the First and the Last, the Beginning and the End."

—Revelation 22:13

Of course, this domino always has ramifications, so we always have choices. The system is designed to give us the choice to move in either a constructive or destructive direction.

Even the smallest detail is not random but the consequence of an exact chain of events. However, some parts of the system are insignificant to the extensive design and not part of the general advancing movement.

As part of the domino system, we may have small freedoms that make no difference in the main direction we are heading. Therefore, some minor details we encounter in life, like choosing the color of a car, may not matter. However, other small details may matter, but we may not know which ones. We may not know which are significant, which are cornerstones, and which are just static noise. As Seneca said: *"Time discovers the truth."*

Becoming human: created in God's image.

Scientific evidence indicates that humans existed millions of years ago. However, the Bible states that humanity may have begun less than ten thousand years ago. Why are there seeming discrepancies between Bible history and what has been found through archeology, fossils, and cave drawings? Evolution indicates that the human brain progressively increased in size as the Earth approached contemporary times. Still, Homo sapiens lived as cave dwellers for millions of years.

Until Adam and Eve received consciousness—or the ability to ask "Why?"—we were not fully human; we were not made in God's image. Instead, humankind was born when God commanded them to avoid eating the forbidden fruit and gave them the choice of whether to obey. This may have occurred only about seven to ten thousand years ago. Before that, we were essentially animals, albeit the most advanced. This is my way of understanding the lack of progress Homo sapiens had until this point in history. There had been many millions of years without significant evolution, without true free mind and free choice. Once we gained consciousness and recognized our Creator's existence, we quickly progressed, becoming more like God. It happened because, with spirituality, our values expanded from just surviving and fleeting self-interest to higher, creative purposes and meanings.

We are responsible for the well-being, nourishment, and enrichment of our souls.

Our physical presence on Earth has the purpose of enriching our eternal soul through the experiences we have in this material world. It is what we leave behind.

This is a beautiful way that God's creations connect to each other and to our souls. It is a way for God to enrich the invisible, eternal world. It transcends time and space as these experiences are transmitted further within the physical as well as spiritual realm.

We are creative lenses for our souls. Having conscious mind and freedom of choice greatly diversifies and enriches these experiences. It can bring us and our souls closer to God. Our material world experiences also connect and make different souls interact with each other when their bodies and minds have and share similar experiences.

But as we know, the mind can be very destructive and damage our souls. That is why we have to work to minimize our natural propensity for damage and enhance our creative, constructive behavior.

We can nourish and enrich our souls more safely when we have experiences that do not typically engage our flesh—experiences like consuming art, meditation or prayer.

As artist Pablo Picasso describes it, *"The purpose of art is washing the dust of daily life off our souls."*

Adopting healthy, constructive habits in following constructive principles is the main way we could achieve this important task.

In summary:

History repeats. It has repeatedly shown that power corrupts, and that human nature does not change regardless of the circumstances. Driven by primitive drives, by greed, pride, and lust, we continue to harm ourselves and others. A new modern culture infiltrated our education and media over the past few decades. It is toxic, as it manipulates our drives and amplifies our natural tendency for abuse. This manifests both at the personal level with the increase in the incidence of chronic diseases and social conflicts and at a large social and geopolitical scale with the creation of a new ideology, a new Marxist-style world order led by the World Economic Forum. This new ideology involves a central global government with a new centralized set of laws and rules "necessary" to address humanity's new "problems" like overpopulation, pandemics, and climate change. To succeed, the new global elite, consisting of most bureaucrats and billionaires in most countries, united by this ideology, uses the same classical techniques of control, but with the help of advanced technology, they are widespread and much more efficient. They have been modifying or deleting our history, old cultural values, and spirituality the same way the communists did last century. In addition, they have been creating crises, conflicts, and chaos at all levels: racial, ethnic, economic, and social. Divide and conquer always worked. Our freedom of speech and other constitutional rights are under threat. They sell your freedom for safety, your health for comfort, and your ancestors' values for the new fairness–equality and "diversity" ideology. You need to open your eyes, wake up, and make the right choices to help revert this evil trend before widespread poverty, violence, and death are unavoidable.

Three perspectives and motivation to change your life.

Whatever book or theory you encounter that addresses health and self-improvement, if you apply the filter that this book offers you, it will help you to distinguish the truth and its value more easily. Applying these three perspectives to the information you receive will help you to filter out the bad from the good:

First: the pre-design perspective and the benefits of match-ing with our body design in whatever we do.

Second: the perspective of being constructive and aligned with the higher purpose of our life, following higher values, detached from immediate worries and conflicts.

And third: the perspective of passing the test of time, and if not matching ancient wisdom, at least not opposing it.

I hope this book will encourage you to change and improve your life. It should motivate and inspire you to discipline yourself and develop good habits to achieve the long-lasting, positive results you long for. Fortunately, you have a significant advantage. You are following the accumulated wisdom of our ancestors and the knowledge of modern science. That is undoubtedly a recipe for success.